T0281671

Hypnotherapy for Pregnancy and Birthing

This practical volume provides resources and guidance for practising hypnotherapy with pregnant women and their birthing partners.

Hypnotherapy for Pregnancy and Birthing begins with an overview of the topic and discusses a range of complex issues and vulnerabilities that might arise during sessions, before moving onto setting up and running group and/or individual sessions. Then, presenting techniques to work with pregnancy and birthing draws on a range of methodologies including solution-focused, metaphors (Ericksonian), Gestalt therapy, benefits approach and regression therapy.

It covers:

- Hypnosis, pregnancy and birthing
- Getting into trance and relaxation
- Breathing
- Practising self-hypnosis and working on issues
- Preparing for birthing
- Bonding with baby
- Working with worries, fears and phobias
- Dealing with trauma and the unexpected
- Loss and bereavement
- Ego boosting.

Containing over 70 customisable scripts and designed to stimulate reflection, this book is a valuable resource for student, newly qualified and experienced hypnotherapists working with pregnancy and birthing.

Jacki Pritchard works as a clinical hypnotherapist, independent social worker and trainer in social care.

Hypnotherapy for Pregnancy and Birthing

Scripts for Hypnotherapists

Jacki Pritchard

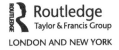

LONDON AND NEW YORK

First published 2022
by Routledge
2 Park Square, Milton Park, Abingdon, Oxon OX14 4RN

and by Routledge
605 Third Avenue, New York, NY 10158

Routledge is an imprint of the Taylor & Francis Group, an informa business

British Library Cataloguing-in-Publication Data
A catalogue record for this book is available from the British Library

Library of Congress Cataloging-in-Publication Data
Names: Pritchard, Jacki, author.
Title: Hypnotherapy for pregnancy and birthing : scripts for hypnotherapists / Jacqueline Pritchard.
Description: Milton Park, Abingdon, Oxon; New York, NY : Routledge, 2021. | Includes bibliographical references and index. | Summary: "This practical volume provides resources and guidance for practising hypnotherapy with pregnant women and their birthing partners. Containing over 40 customisable scripts and designed to stimulate reflection, this book is a valuable resource for both beginner and experienced hypnotherapists working with pregnancy and birth"—Provided by publisher.
Identifiers: LCCN 2021005381 (print) | LCCN 2021005382 (ebook) | ISBN 9781032003504 (hardback) | ISBN 9781032003498 (paperback) | ISBN 9781003173779 (ebook)
Subjects: LCSH: Pregnancy. | Childbirth. | Hypnotism–Therapeutic use.
Classification: LCC RG551.P757 2021 (print) | LCC RG551 (ebook) | DDC 618.2—dc23
LC record available at https://lccn.loc.gov/2021005381
LC ebook record available at https://lccn.loc.gov/2021005382

ISBN: 978-1-032-00350-4 (hbk)
ISBN: 978-1-032-00349-8 (pbk)
ISBN: 978-1-003-17377-9 (ebk)

DOI: 10.4324/9781003173779

Typeset in Times New Roman
by codeMantra

This book is dedicated in memoriam to Mary Sarjeant who taught me about 'true rest' and 'nourishing change'.

Contents

PART I
Hypnosis, pregnancy and birthing   1

1 Using hypnosis for pregnancy and birthing: understanding
   vulnerabilities and complexities   3

2 How to use the book and scripts   12

3 The importance of assessment and evaluation   21
   Appendix 3.1: Assessment questionnaire for a pregnancy
   and birthing group 24
   Appendix 3.2: Example of a standard consent form 25

4 Running a group   27
   Appendix 4.1: Summary of essential questions 36

5 Individual sessions   37

PART II
Getting into trance and relaxation   43

6 The rainbow scarf   45

7 The hypno mat   48

8 Marshmallows   51

9 Counting watermelon seeds   53

PART III
Breathing   55

10 Breathing   57

11 Visualisations   62

12 Fanning out   69
Script 1: The peacock 69
Script 2: The flamenco dancer's fan 70

13 Breathing with the waves   72
Additional script 1: Waving goodbye to morning sickness 75

14 Going skiing   76

15 Flying high in a plane   79

16 Let's imagine water   82
Additional script 1: Birthing pool 83
Additional script 2: Pond 83
Additional script 3: Fountain in the ground 83
Additional script 4: Waterfall 84
Additional script 5: Water park 84

PART IV
Practising self-hypnosis and working on issues   87

17 The practice nest   89

18 Dad: you're important too   91

19 Exercising in the gym   95
Additional script 1: Taking a stretch class 96
Additional script 2: Personal trainer 97
Additional script 3: Lifting weights 98
Additional script 4: Pedalling time away 98

20 The bathroom   100

21 The healing place   104
*Additional script 1: Swooshing and cleansing for
   nausea/morning sickness 106*

22 Body scanner   107
Additional script 1: Talking with baby 109

23 Tunnel of calmness   111
   Additional script 1: Meeting baby 114
   Additional script 2: The half white circle gauge 114

24 Sleeping blankets   116

25 Your very own hotel   119
   Additional script 1: The lower floor – the past 120
   Additional script 2: The first floor – the future 122

PART V
Preparing for birthing   125

26 Be prepared   127
   Additional script 1: The nursery 128
   Additional script 2: Packing a bag 129
   Additional script 3: Material things do not matter 131

27 Birthing plan   132
   Appendix 27.1: Questionnaire for developing a birthing plan 135

28 A trip to the cinema   136

29 Journey to the hospital   138
   Script 1: For mum 138
   Script 2: For dad/birthing partner 141

30 Birthing room   145
   Script 1: Hospital setting – for mum 145
   Script 2: Hospital setting – for dad/birthing partner 148

31 Birthing at home   151
   Script 1: For mum 151
   Script 2: For dad/birthing partner 154

PART VI
Bonding with baby   157

32 Bonding on the beach   159

33 Message room   162
   Additional script 1: The message jar 163
   Additional script 2: Welcome messages for baby 164
   Additional script 3: A bit of graffiti 165
   Additional script 4: Message board for affirmations 166
   Additional script 5: Recording what you want to say 167
   Additional script 6: Keeping a journal 169

34 Portfolio of perfect photographs   170

PART VII
Working with worries, fears and phobias   175

35 The old mining village   177
   Additional script 1: The churchyard 178
   Additional script 2: The well dressing 179
   Additional script 3: The pit 180

36 Ice sculpture   182

37 The book of untruths   184

PART VIII
Dealing with trauma and the unexpected   189

38 It is your body   191

39 Distraction   193
   Additional script 1: Dealing with the unexpected 195
   Additional script 2: The wall 196

40 The shadow   197

PART IX
Loss and bereavement   199

41 Loss and bereavement   201

42 The angels' archway   205

43 Letting go of baby   208

PART X
Ego boosting   211

44 The emotional flowerpot   213

45 Superwoman   216

46 The rocky mountain   219

47 You can so do this   222

48 The ballerina   224

49 Sadie   227

50 Well done you   230

    Index   233

Part I

Hypnosis, pregnancy and birthing

1 Using hypnosis for pregnancy and birthing
Understanding vulnerabilities and complexities

Introduction

The main objective of this book is to present scripts which will help a hypnotherapist (or hypnobirthing teacher) to use hypnosis effectively for pregnancy and birthing. I have written this book specifically for hypnotherapists – whether they are training, newly qualified or experienced. I am writing with two hats on: as a clinical hypnotherapist who enjoys working with pregnancy and birthing but also as a social worker who has supported many pregnant people over the years when they have needed help with complex problems. This is the reason why I wanted to look at pregnancy and birthing from a wider perspective. In all my years working as a social worker I have learnt that very often the problem a client presents with is not actually the main issue. Sometimes it can take time for the underlying problem to come to the surface. It is exactly the same when practising hypnotherapy. A client can contact a hypnotherapist for help with something specific and then once the treatment plan is in place and therapy is underway, the subconscious mind reveals related or other problems. A pregnant mum (and dad/birthing partner) could be attending a group or an individual session to learn breathing and relaxation techniques, but other issues are identified.

Using hypnosis is a really effective therapeutic tool to help mum with her pregnancy and prepare her for the birth using any number of techniques. The use of self-hypnosis can be extremely beneficial to mum and anyone else who might be going to support her. There are very many books written about pregnancy and childbirth and, since the 1980s, hypnobirthing has become very popular and trendy amongst certain sections of some societies. This is a very good thing, but the texts are often limited in that they do not consider the wider issues and problems that already exist for a client or those which can come to light during a pregnancy.

This book goes beyond what has become known as hypnobirthing and raises awareness about issues, problems and situations which could be presented to a hypnotherapist. I wanted to look beyond the stereotypical pregnant woman or couple. I want hypnotherapists to think about who their pregnant (or pregnant-related) clients might be:

- Child, young person or adult
- Mum (who could be in a one-parent situation or in a relationship)
- Biological dad
- A partner (i.e. in a relationship with mum but not the biological father of the baby)
- Surrogate
- Intended parents

DOI: 10.4324/9781003173779-1

- Birthing partner
- Couples: heterosexual, gay, lesbian, transgender, non-binary.

The book will help hypnotherapists to facilitate pregnancy and birthing groups and individual sessions, which will be beneficial to pregnant clients in general; but in addition the book raises awareness about important societal issues and the vulnerability of some clients which can result in complex cases.

History and developments

For an excessively long time, childbirth was seen very much as a medical matter and clinical procedures dominated the birth of the baby. In the twentieth century, some parts of the world became more enlightened. In the UK during the 1920s it was a doctor who first started thinking differently about childbirth and about the use of hypnosis in pregnancy. Grantly Dick-Read worked as an obstetrician and used the term 'natural childbirth', which was the title of his first book, *Natural Childbirth*.[1] Another book he wrote, *Childbirth without Fear*, which was originally written in 1942, is still available and well worth reading.[2] The term 'hypnobirthing' became popular in the 1980s and since then the use of hypnobirthing methods has developed worldwide. For someone who wants to focus solely on hypnobirthing techniques, I think it is useful to read the latest versions of the well-established texts written by Michelle Leclaire O' Neill,[3] Marie Mongan[4] and Katharine Graves.[5] A hypnobirthing teacher will normally follow a particular method (e.g. the Leclaire method,[6] the Mongan method[7] or the KGH method[8]) and may provide a book about the method as part of the hypnobirthing package they offer. The original texts, in some way, are presented like self-help books so are a helpful resource after the group classes have finished.

Hypnobirthing has become more and more popular during the past 40 years and women certainly now have more say in where and how they want to give birth. Quite rightly so after centuries of being told what to do (and what is best for them) by physicians, nurses and midwives. I welcome the progress that has been made as I totally believe it is a basic human right that a mum should decide how she wants to go through her pregnancy and ultimately deliver her baby. I am not forgetting dads in all of this but will come to them later. Suffice to say they have rights too.

It must be acknowledged that at the time of writing this book the ongoing Covid-19 pandemic has affected how services are delivered to pregnant women and their birthing partners. Women have had to face many things alone and consequently have felt isolated and unsupported. Some midwives feel that choices have been limited for women giving birth and it is as though steps have been taken backwards.

Being properly qualified

In any profession it is imperative to undergo thorough training to develop knowledge and skills in order to become properly qualified, that is, fully equipped to do the job. It is also important that, once qualified, a professional continues to undergo training for their own professional development in order to maintain best practice. All this is true for a hypnotherapist, who should be trained by a reputable training school so that they can join a professional body and then undertake the required hours for Continued Professional Development (CPD).

When something becomes popular, people tend to hop on the bandwagon. With hypnobirthing, some people who want to run groups and classes may attend one or more taster sessions, learn some techniques and then believe they can teach others. They have learnt the hypnobirthing theory, concepts and techniques but many are not properly qualified as a hypnotherapist or hypnobirthing teacher. There are many professionals who do become hypnobirthing teachers and are not hypnotherapists (e.g. nurses in GP surgeries; midwives) and are well-equipped to deliver hypnobirthing groups. I feel strongly that in order to run any groups professionally and effectively, some basic training in group work is also needed.[9]

It is a fact that hypnosis is a natural state and we all go into trance at least one hundred times a day. The subconscious mind can take a person to different places – very often unexpectedly but with a purpose. The subconscious mind knows when things need to be addressed and worked on. People who are not properly qualified as a hypnotherapist may not know what to do when someone abreacts, that is, releases a suppressed memory – maybe of a traumatic event – and the emotions associated with it. This is when the skills of a properly qualified hypnotherapist are needed.

Anyone who wants to provide hypnosis for pregnancy and birthing should undertake some specialist training. A hypnotherapist might do this as part of their CPD. I believe that a hypnotherapist can offer so much more than just hypnobirthing techniques and from my own experience I think this is what is often needed. Common problems the hypnotherapist may have to deal with when working with pregnancy and birthing are:

- Lack of confidence/assertiveness; self-doubt; low self esteem
- Anxiety
- Fears/phobias
- Intrusive/obsessive thoughts and feelings
- Relationship problems
- Isolation (lack of support)
- Long-term effects of: bullying; neglect; abuse
- Trust issues
- Health issues (physical and/or mental).

The hypnotherapist will be able to use and transfer methods of working and specific techniques they know and already use in their day-to-day practice. It is beneficial to use a registered hypnotherapist to help with pregnancy and birthing because they will have:

- Proper training and qualifications in hypnotherapy
- Specialist training in pregnancy and birthing
- Knowledge
- Skills
- Techniques
- The ability to develop packages/treatment plans.

Safety issues

Another concern of mine is that it is very easy to find hypnobirthing groups being advertised on the internet. For some groups it is possible for people to sign up on online and then just turn up for a class. No proper assessment is undertaken beforehand. Before using hypnosis, it is crucial to know if a client has any physical or mental health problems, is taking any medication, has any particular fears or phobias. In order to obtain this information, it is best practice to undertake a thorough assessment, which is discussed in Chapter 3. Hypnotherapists cannot treat people who have certain conditions, such as, psychosis or epilepsy (although there are different views about hypnotherapists treating epilepsy; some insurance companies can refuse to cover a hypnotherapist who works with a client who has been diagnosed with this condition).

I also worry about the health and safety of the hypnotherapist. I believe screening is very important especially when doing group work to ensure the safety of the hypnotherapist and group members (e.g. when running a group for pregnant girls who are in care and may present with many different types of behaviours; or for women who have been force married and may be watched or followed by members of their family or community). The hypnotherapist may need to obtain some background information from other professionals/workers to ensure they and other members of the group are not at risk of harm in any way due to violence or behavioural problems, such as, someone misusing drugs or alcohol. There are so many things to think about before working with a group of people (see Chapter 4).

When pregnancy is not good news

Women have been giving birth for thousands of years; it is one of the most natural things to do all around the world. It should be one of the most wonderful experiences in anyone's lifetime whether you are a mum or a dad. The reality is that when something is supposed to be a wonderful, good or positive experience sometimes it is not. A bad experience can affect people – how they think, feel and behave – for both short and long periods of time. The expectations of society, communities, families, friends and other individuals can put undue emotional pressure on a person. Pregnancy and the birth of a baby are supposed to be good news events, but for some they are not.

There are many books about hypnobirthing that give a lot of good information and I think they can be an excellent resource for practising techniques which have been taught. However, I think a lot of important issues are often not addressed. I have been a social worker for over four decades and have worked with a lot of pregnant young girls and women (and men, i.e. biological dads) during that time. Pregnancy is not always welcomed or situations arise which cause a lot of problems. The reality is for some girls and women it can be the worst news they have ever received. Some of the situations in which a female might not want to be pregnant are (and this list is not exhaustive by any means):

- Very young girl becomes pregnant (the youngest pregnant girl I have known was 11 years old)
- Pregnant as a result of a one-night stand
- Not knowing who the dad is
- Pregnant after being raped
- The baby is the product of sexual abuse/incestuous relationship/forced marriage
- Currently living in a domestic abuse situation
- Dad of the baby finishes the relationship after hearing about the pregnancy
- Dad does not want to be a parent/does not want/like children at all
- Dad already has children and does not want any more.

Common fears

People do not suddenly stop having other issues or problems when they become pregnant. I believe wholeheartedly that positivity is something which should be promoted in any therapeutic work which is being undertaken. Hypnobirthing books do promote a positive attitude to pregnancy and natural childbirth, especially in regard to the use of language, but few address the practical or emotional issues which some pregnant people may be facing – and I definitely think it should be acknowledged that dads can have the same worries as mums. Some common fears are:

- Having a miscarriage
- Not going full-term
- Stillbirth
- Something being wrong with the baby
- Not having any feelings for the baby when s/he arrives
- The actual birth
- Not being able to be a good parent
- Not being able to cope.

Hypnobirthing texts may talk about fear at some level, but very often specific fears and phobias which have been an issue for a long time, need to be worked on, such as:

- Fear of being physically sick
- Fainting at the sight of blood
- Phobia regarding needles.

Hypnobirthing texts do acknowledge that fear is something that has to be dealt with and the theory is that by learning and practising hypnobirthing techniques, mum is going to become relaxed and calm. I totally agree with this, but feel that some fears cannot be dealt with in-depth in a group/class setting. Very often it requires individual sessions with mum (or dad/birthing partner) to work on whatever the issues are. In my own practice the most common issues I have had to work with during individual hypnotherapy sessions have been:

- Fear of history repeating itself:
  - relative died in childbirth
  - parent was abusive, so they will be (due to the belief it is genetic)
- Habits/addictions:
  - smoking
  - alcohol
  - drugs
- History of abuse or currently living in an abusive situation:
  - fear for own/baby's safety
  - lack of confidence
  - low self-esteem
  - feeling of worthlessness.

A person's past and what is embedded in their subconscious mind affect who they are today – how they think, feel and behave. Current fears can stem from the past or some can be brought to the forefront of the subconscious mind because of the pregnancy. Something which has happened in the past may have been suppressed and not dealt with. So, regression work can be a useful method to use.

Vulnerability and complex cases

It is vital to be person-centred when delivering hypnotherapy to any client but I want to highlight the fact that so many societal issues can come into play when working with pregnancy and birthing. Some readers might think some of the topics or situations I mention below would not be pertinent to a hypnotherapist and I am only raising them because I also practise as a social worker. However, all sorts of people seek help from a hypnotherapist. Clients can come from all walks of life and backgrounds; there is no stereotypical hypnotherapy client. Therefore, I think a hypnotherapist has to have some awareness and knowledge about the following in order to be prepared to help clients with pregnancy and birthing:

- Child abuse[10]
- Adult abuse[11]
- Sexual abuse
- Domestic violence (both female and male victims)
- Forced marriage and honour-based violence[12]
- Modern slavery (domestic servitude and human trafficking).[13]

I have separated out sexual abuse from the other categories of abuse to make the important point that any person who has been sexually abused may not like to be touched in any way at all (even a simple handshake or a pat on the arm). The prospect of having to be medically examined through her pregnancy and during birthing could raise many issues and worries for a female victim.

Some common fears were discussed earlier, but a victim of abuse may have more specific fears, which the hypnotherapist needs to understand. The list below may seem extreme but any one of the fears could be very real for a victim who has had horrendous things done to them in the past. A victim could have a specific fear of:

- Being found if they have escaped from an abusive situation, e.g. by their abuser; family member or someone from the community (if a victim of forced marriage); gangmaster/lieutenant (if a victim of modern slavery)
- Punishment
- Violence
- Death
- Being locked in somewhere (having have been incarcerated previously – perhaps for long periods of time)
- Never being able to return home
- Being sent abroad
- Family members being threatened/harmed/murdered
- Anyone in a position of authority
- Being convicted of a crime (having been forced to commit crimes by their abuser).

Historical abuse may be disclosed by mum or it may be seen/talked about when mum is in trance, that is, the subconscious mind may take her to a traumatic/abusive incident.

Alternatively, mum could be living in an abusive situation currently. The hypnotherapist may pick up the signs from the way mum or her partner behave and will face the dilemma regarding reporting and breaking confidentiality. This is why confidentiality always needs to be discussed at length before hypnotherapy starts. Any hypnotherapist needs to undertake some basic awareness training in regard to safeguarding children and safeguarding adults. The policies and procedures are different for children and adults because of the legislation which exists[14] and the related statutory guidance.[15] It is useful for the hypnotherapist to try to attend the basic awareness courses provided their local authority, details of which should be available via the websites for the local Safeguarding Partnership (for children) and Safeguarding Adults Board.[16]

If a mum or dad/partner is known to Children's Social Care or Adult Social Care, then the hypnotherapist could be asked to attend meetings, reviews and possibly have a role in plans which are developed for a mum, existing child or future baby. If a pre-birth assessment is being undertaken, the hypnotherapist could be asked for their opinion if they are working with a mum, dad or partner. Another scenario could be that a young girl who is in care becomes pregnant. The hypnotherapist could work with the girl either because they are asked to do so by Children's Social Care or because they are referred by a school in which the hypnotherapist works. Hence, a simple referral for hypnosis to help with pregnancy and birthing can become a complex case.

Other important issues which a hypnotherapist needs to have some knowledge about and understanding are:

- *Homelessness*: a misconception is that hypnotherapists will only be seeing clients who can afford to pay for therapy. The reality is that hypnotherapists may be commissioned by organisations or some choose to work pro bono in some circumstances in order to give something back to the community. Therefore, the hypnotherapist could work with a mum who is homeless or has been in the past.
- *Poverty*: a young girl or woman could be living in poverty whilst being pregnant and be very concerned about her future. Or mum may have experienced poverty earlier in life and has a fear that she could find herself in such circumstances again. Mums who have previously been neglected can binge-eat even when there is no shortage of food or they can develop eating disorders.
- *Equality, diversity and discrimination*: all professionals/workers should undertake some training about equality and diversity and have an understanding of the *Equality Act* 2010.[17] We like to think that the majority of professionals/workers practise in a non-discriminatory way, but the reality is some do not and in fact some can be very judgemental. It is against the law to discriminate against anyone because of:

  - age
  - gender reassignment
  - being married or in a civil partnership
  - being pregnant or on maternity leave
  - disability
  - race including colour, nationality, ethnic or national origin
  - religion or belief
  - sex
  - sexual orientation.

- *Gender identity*: sensitivity is needed in this area of work as knowledge increases and language changes. The hypnotherapist could find themselves working with a transgender dad or non-binary individual who is pregnant.
- *Surrogacy*: the hypnotherapist could work with a surrogate and the intended parents and needs to have some knowledge of the legalities of surrogacy.
- *Loss and bereavement*: so many different types of loss (not just death) can be experienced through childhood and into adulthood, some of which may not have been dealt with, or memories and feelings are brought to the forefront when mum becomes pregnant (not just for mum but other people in her life too).

These topics will be mentioned through the book when introducing the scripts, but the hypnotherapist or hypnobirthing teacher should really think about their level of knowledge and whether they need to read around a more specialised subject area or seek in-depth training. The hypnotherapist can research topics, but I think it is important to undertake proper training (face-to-face courses or webinars) and plan this as part of their CPD. It may not be possible to find appropriate training immediately but it may be something the hypnotherapist will identify as an area for training in the future. I make some suggestions regarding books and useful websites within the chapters. The following chapter explains how the book is presented and how the hypnotherapist can find their way around it and locate a script they need.

Notes

1 Dick-Read, G. (1933) *Natural Childbirth* (no longer in print).
2 Dick-Read, G. (2004) *Childbirth without Fear.* London: Pinter and Martin Ltd.
3 O'Neill, M.L. (2019) *Hypnobirthing: the original method.* Pacific Palisades, CA: Papyrus Press.
4 Mongan, M. (2016) *Hypnobirthing the Mongan Method: the breakthrough approach to safer, easier, comfortable birthing.* 4th edition. London: Souvenir Press.
5 Graves, K. (2017) *The Hypnobirthing Book: An inspirational guide for a calm, confident, natural birth.* 2nd edition. Marlborough, Wiltshire: Katharine Publishing.
6 https://www.leclairemethod.com/.
7 https://us.hypnobirthing.com/.
8 https://www.kghypnobirthing.com/.
9 Some older texts on group work are well worth reading as a starting point: Doel, M. and Sawdon, C. (1999) *The Essential Groupworker: Teaching and learning creative group work.* London: Jessica Kingsley Publishers; Douglas, T. (2000) *Basic Groupwork* (2nd edition). London: Tavistock Publications Ltd.
10 There are four categories of child abuse under the *Children Act 1989*: physical abuse; sexual abuse; emotional abuse and neglect.
11 There are ten forms of abuse under the *Care Act 2014*: physical abuse; domestic violence; sexual abuse; psychological abuse; financial/material abuse; modern slavery; discriminatory abuse; organisational abuse; neglect/act of omission; self-neglect.
12 The hypnotherapist who has little knowledge about forced marriage may find it helpful to read as a general introduction: HM Government (June 2014) *Multi-agency Practice Guidelines: Handling Cases of Forced Marriage.* https://assets.publishing.service.gov.uk/government/uploads/system/uploads/attachment_data/file/322307/HMG_MULTI_AGENCY_PRACTICE_GUIDELINES_v1_180614_FINAL.pdf.
13 A useful introduction to modern slavery is: HM Government (November 2014) *Modern Slavery Strategy* and a useful report on developments since 2015 is: The Centre for Social Justice/Justice and Care, *It Still Happens Here: Fighting UK Slavery in the 2020s.* London: Justice and Care. https://www.justiceandcare.org/wp-content/uploads/2020/07/Justice-and-Care-Centre-for-Social-Justice-It-Still-Happens-Here.pdf.

14 In England, safeguarding children work is legislated by *the Children Act 1989* and *Children Act 2004*. Safeguarding adults work is legislated by the *Care Act 2014*. Other legislation exists for other parts of Great Britain, i.e., Wales, Scotland and Northern Ireland.
15 In England: HM Government (April 2018) *Working Together to Safeguard Children: A guide to inter-agency working to safeguard and promote the welfare of children*. For adults: Care and Support Statutory Guidance to be found at: https://www.gov.uk/government/publications/care-act-statutory-guidance/care-and-support-statutory-guidance.
16 These can be found by going to a local authority's website in the first instance.
17 It can be useful to read the guidance that goes with the act; this can be found at: https://www.gov.uk/guidance/equality-act-2010-guidance.

2   How to use the book and scripts

I wanted this book to be a very practical resource for hypnotherapists by including an abundance of tried and tested scripts. It is essential that a hypnotherapist using the book can find their way around it easily and quickly locate an appropriate script for their work. So, I have divided the book into sections, which is a logical progression through subject areas and themes which might be covered in a pregnancy and birthing group or in individual sessions. Below I shall briefly summarise the main objective of each section and then provide a key to the scripts. Some of the scripts have one main objective; others will serve more than one purpose and could in fact have been put in several sections.

Using the scripts

The scripts offer a variety of methodology to choose from:

- Solution-focussed
- Metaphors (Ericksonian)
- Gestalt therapy
- Benefits approach
- Regression.

Where scripts are included in a chapter, there is an introduction to explain their purpose and how they can be used – either for group work or individual sessions. Some scripts need more in-depth explanation; consequently a number of introductions are longer than others. In several chapters, additional short scripts follow a main script. The hypnotherapist will interpret the script and present it in their own way, that is, choose their own intonation, pauses and silences as they work with and respond to a client or group. I have included *guidance notes* and suggested prompts/questions, within the body of the scripts.

   Some of the scripts are suitable and intended for use by dad/birthing partner during the birthing process. In my own practice I sometimes give out a script during a session (group or individual) so dad/birthing partner can practise at home.

Use of language

One of the main things taught in hypnobirthing is about the use of language. The objective being to get away from the medical model and old-fashioned terminology. I do not disagree with any of it and when I am focussed solely on teaching hypnobirthing

DOI: 10.4324/9781003173779-2

techniques, I teach the hypnobirthing language as well. The following examples are taken from the Mongan method[1]:

Traditional language	Hypnobirthing alternative
Contraction	Uterine surge or wave
Coach	Birth champion
Catch the baby	Receive the baby
Deliver/delivery	Birth/birthing
Due date	Birthing time/month
Pain/contractions	Pressure/sensation tightening
Water breaking/rupturing	Membrane release
Birth canal	Birth path
Pushing	Birth breathing
Complications	Special circumstances
Mucous plug	Uterine seal
Bloody show	Birth show
Transition	Near completion/nearly complete
Effacing/dilating	Thinning/opening
Foetus	Pre-born/unborn baby
Primip/multip	First/second-time mum
Perineal rim stretches	Perineal rim unfolds
Clients/patients	Parents
Braxton-Hicks	Pre-labour warm ups
Kegels	Pelvic floor exercises
Neonate	New born
Stalled/shut-down labour	Resting labour
False labour	Practise labour

However, for some clients the hypnobirthing language just does not feel right to them. For example, a 15-year-old girl might prefer to use the term 'contraction' rather than 'wave' or 'surge'. These latter terms can often elicit giggles from a group of young girls, who think the words are 'posh' or 'hippyish'. I like to work in a person-centred way, so if I am going to use a variety of methods, I have a discussion about language and let the client develop their own preferred language – use of words and phrases – as we work together over the sessions.

In this book, for simplicity, I use the terms:

- Mum (to cover any pregnant person whether a child, adult, surrogate, transgender man, non-binary individual)
- Dad (biological)
- Intended parents (parents who may be using a surrogate)
- Birthing partner (if someone other than dad is going to help mum at the birth)
- Birthing (for childbirth)
- Pregnancy and birthing group
- Group session (i.e. class run for a pregnancy and birthing group)
- Individual session (i.e. rather than a group session; such sessions are conducted for one person or a couple, or possibly a trio if there is a surrogate and intended parents).

Face-to-face sessions and working remotely

I started thinking about this book and putting it together before the Covid-19 pandemic started to affect our lives and the world at large. The year 2020 was like no other – offering many challenges for all professionals and certainly hypnotherapists, many of whom have chosen to work remotely when they have not been able to work face-to-face with clients. The book has been written based on the idea of working face-to-face with clients. However, many of the issues discussed and the scripts included in the text will be of use to hypnotherapists who continue to work remotely in the future. All I want to emphasise is what good practitioners should know already – safety and confidentiality have to be of paramount importance and extra care and assessment need to be undertaken before delivering a session via the internet. It is imperative that hypnotherapists follow (and keep up to date with) guidance from their professional bodies and insurers.

The parts

What follows is a brief summary of what each part in the book covers.

I Hypnosis, pregnancy and birthing

This introductory part discusses the historical developments in using hypnosis to work with pregnancy and birthing and current approaches (group work and individual sessions) and introduces a recurring theme through the book – the importance of assessment and evaluation.

II Getting into trance and relaxation

The scripts in this part are for use in a first session (group or individual). They can be used to introduce the client (mum, dad/birthing partner or others) to hypnosis, the trance state and demonstrate the power of the imagination. One of the main objectives is for the client to experience true relaxation.

III Breathing

This part aims to discuss the importance of learning to breathe and then teach a variety of breathing techniques for use during pregnancy and for birthing. The concept of the birthing journey is introduced by using specific hypnobirthing techniques – up and down breathing; stretching muscles; opening the cervix and the birthing.

IV Practising self-hypnosis and working on issues

This part offers different places where the client can practice self-hypnosis and the new techniques they learn in each session. Some of the places can be created as a 'safe place' but primarily they are places for practising. Work can begin on particular issues/problems and many of the scripts can be returned to in future sessions to develop the work further.

V Preparing for birthing

The word 'preparation' is just as important as 'practise' when working with pregnancy and birthing. This part includes scripts which help the client to focus on what needs to be done in a practical sense during the pregnancy and to prepare for the actual birthing (whether it be in hospital or at home).

VI Bonding with baby

Very simply the scripts in this part include many different ways to bond with a baby, which is such an important aspect of the work to be undertaken.

VII Working with worries, fears and phobias

The scripts are designed specifically to work on any worries mum, dad or birthing partner may be experiencing – from a simple worry to something more serious which has been affecting him/her for some time, that is, before the pregnancy.

VIII Dealing with trauma and the unexpected

The scripts in this part are specifically for mums who, as a consequence of having experienced abuse or other trauma in their life, may find medical examinations intrusive; they might not like to be touched and would find any unexpected procedure harrowing.

IX Loss and bereavement

Being pregnant can bring up issues for a client related to different types of loss and also bereavement. Sometimes a client thinks they have dealt with a loss or death from the past but the pregnancy resurrects memories, regrets, unhelpful feelings or fears. Future losses are also addressed.

X Ego boosting

All the scripts in this part offer ways of working on lack of confidence, low self-esteem and self-doubt. Although this part comes at the end of the book, the scripts within it can be used in earlier sessions as issues are worked on. The final chapter is for use in the last session in order to commend mum and reinforce positivity.

Guide to the chapters/scripts

The guide should be used to find an appropriate script/subject area.

1	Using hypnosis for pregnancy and birthing: understanding vulnerabilities and complexities	*Historical perspective; being qualified; safety issues; when pregnancy is not good news; common fears; vulnerable clients; abuse*
2	How to use the book and scripts	
3	The importance of assessment and evaluation *Appendix 3.1: Assessment questionnaire for a pregnancy and birthing group* *Appendix 3.2: Example of a standard consent form*	*Discussion about how assessments should be undertaken; value of evaluating*

(Continued)

4 Running a group   *Discussion and questions in order to plan, set up and run a pregnancy and birthing group*

Appendix 4.1: Summary of essential questions

5 Individual sessions   *Discussion around working with individuals, different types of couples/trios (e.g. surrogates and intended parents)*

6 The rainbow scarf   *Introduction to trance; deep relaxation; use for self-hypnosis*

7 The hypno mat   *Demonstrates the power of the imagination; taking control; travelling for distraction; creating a safe place; emphasises and promotes the importance of wellbeing; a place to practise in future sessions*

8 Marshmallows   *A way of getting into trance; deepener; the big marshmallow can be used as a safe place*

9 Counting watermelon seeds   *Visualisation; relaxation; counting down into trance*

10 Breathing   *Discussion about the importance of initially teaching basic breathing techniques: number, ratio and colour breathing*

11 Visualisations   *To develop effective breathing (up and down) and distraction techniques. Can be read by dad/birthing partner to help mum practise and during birthing*

12 Fanning out   *To facilitate the opening of the cervix for birthing*
   Script 1: The peacock
   Script 2: The flamenco dancer's fan

13 Breathing with the waves *a*   *Relaxation. To practise breathing techniques; teaches continuous, smooth breathing for birthing*

   Additional script 1: Waving goodbye to morning sickness   *Breathing away nausea/sickness*

14 Going skiing   *To promote the concept of a journey for birthing. To practise up and down breathing*

15 Flying high in a plane   *To promote the concept of a journey for birthing. To practise up and down breathing*

16 Let's imagine water   *Relaxation and getting into trance using water as a visualisation in different locations*

   Additional script 1: Birthing pool   *Visualisation. Forward pacing to the birthing journey. Exploring the pool. Who should be present. Changing the temperature of the water*

   Additional script 2: Pond   *Relaxation and promoting smooth movement*

   Additional script 3: Fountain in the ground   *Cooling down body temperature. To feel refreshed and energised*

   Additional script 4: Waterfall   *Cooling down*

   Additional script 5: Water park   *Cooling down. Relaxation. Deepener. Making time pass quickly. Bonding with baby and forward pacing*

17 The practice nest   *To create a specific place where mum can practise self-hypnosis regularly. Can be returned to in future sessions for use in conjunction with other scripts*

18 Dad: You're important too — *Specific script for dad using the benefits approach to relax; practise breathing; focus on remaining calm; considers dad's role and responsibilities*

19 Exercising in the gym — *To focus on exercising and being healthy. Motivation and determination. Breathing. Can be returned to in future sessions*

   Additional script 1: Taking a stretch class — *Breathing and stretching in preparation for birthing*

   Additional script 2: Personal trainer — *Connecting with the subconscious mind (the trainer) to work on issues in future sessions. A key objective is for the trainer to help with motivation*

   Additional script 3: Lifting weights — *To get rid of a worry, concern or fear*

   Additional script 4: Pedalling time away — *To make time pass more quickly*

20 The bathroom — *Relaxation. Deepening. For practising down breathing. A place to get rid of things, e.g. thought, feeling or fear. Embeds positive thoughts and way of thinking. Comfort and protection. Stretching for birthing*

21 The healing place — *Healing (physically or emotionally). Ideal as a safe place. Relaxation. Restoring energy*

   Additional script 1: Swooshing and cleansing for nausea/morning sickness

22 Body scanner — *Working on physical and/or emotional problems. Analysis of perception i.e. how the client views a problem and then works on it*

   Additional script 1: Talking with baby — *Bonding*

23 Tunnel of calmness — *Working on high blood pressure. Relaxation and calmness*

   Additional script 1: Meeting baby — *Bonding*

   Additional script 2: The half white circle gauge — *Reducing high blood pressure*

24 Sleeping blankets — *To work on any sleeping difficulties being experienced in pregnancy. Can be used for rest periods during the birthing journey; and for after the baby is born when mum needs to sleep*

25 Your very own hotel — *A place to relax; be safe; have fun; for practise. To work on the past, present or future and related issues*

   Additional script 1: The lower floor (the past) — *Regression technique to find the root cause of a problem*

   Additional script 2: The first floor (the future) — *To work on the future: preparation, planning and forward pacing*

26 Be prepared — *Preparations during pregnancy; for the client to identify what needs to be done before the birth. Particularly good for clients who are not very organised*

(Continued)

Additional script 1: The nursery

Additional script 2: Packing a bag

Additional script 3: Material things do not matter — Particularly designed for clients who may be living in poverty/struggling financially and are worried about providing for the baby

27 Birthing plan — To develop a birthing plan which includes what mum needs; what she wants to happen (or things which should not be done or said) but also to include: relevant history; background information; significant experiences; fears or worries

Appendix 27.1: Questionnaire for developing a birthing plan

28 A trip to the cinema — Creates the cinema for forward pacing: planning how things should happen; rehearsal and embedding. To be used in conjunction with the following three chapters

29 Journey to the hospital — Forward pacing

Script 1: For mum

Script 2: For a birthing partner

30 Birthing room — Forward pacing

Script 1: Hospital setting – for mum

Script 2: Hospital setting – for a birthing partner

31 Birthing at home — Forward pacing

Script 1: For mum

Script 2: For a birthing partner

32 Bonding on the beach — A specific place for mum to bond with baby on a regular basis – taking time for self. Relaxation. Deepener

33 Message room — Creates a specific room to communicate with the baby and encourage bonding. To be used in conjunction with the following scripts which facilitate communication (with the baby and other people) by talking, writing, drawing and recording

Additional script 1: The message jar — To create and keep messages

Additional script 2: Welcome messages — To create welcome messages for when the baby arrives

Additional script 3: A bit of graffiti — To affirm beliefs and positive thoughts using words and phrases

Additional script 4: Message board for affirmations — To create affirmations

Additional script 5: Recording what you want to say — Exploring and expressing thoughts/feelings. Rehearsal for difficult conversations/situations (e.g. with relatives, friends or professionals)

Additional script 6: Keeping a journal	*A place to recall and store positive memories of the pregnancy. Can also be used to work on past events, incidents related to a specific concern or fear*
34 Portfolio of perfect photographs	*To focus mum (or dad) on how she wants things to be in the future. Embeds the ability to experiment, make changes and adjustments to get things just right*
35 The old mining village	*To get rid of anything that is preventing mum (or anyone else) from enjoying the pregnancy. The following three scripts provide different locations to get rid of fears, memories (e.g. previous bad birthing experience) and release emotions*
Additional script 1: The churchyard	
Additional script 2: The well dressing	
Additional script 3: The pit	
36 Ice sculpture	*Dealing with any fear from the past (childhood, adolescence or adulthood) or a fear which develops in relation to the pregnancy or birthing (e.g. dad's fear of passing out at the sight of blood/needles)*
37 The book of untruths	*To work on self-doubt, low self-esteem and lack of confidence, which have stemmed from things said and done in the past. Particularly good for working with survivors of child/adult abuse or domestic violence. To focus on how to be more assertive and expressing oneself (using words and phrases; and rehearsal)*
38 It is your body	*Particularly for mums who do not like being looked at or touched due to past trauma and for whom medical examinations or unexpected procedures could become another traumatic event for them*
39 Distraction	*To reinforce what has been learnt in earlier sessions regarding using hypnosis for distraction. Introduces new methods of travelling. Can be used by dad/birthing partner to support mum during an unexpected procedure*
Additional script 1: Dealing with the unexpected	*For dad/birthing partner to read to mum when forceps are used; she has to have stitches or she is told a caesarean is necessary*
Additional script 2: The wall	*To help mum detach from what is being done to her physically*
40 The shadow	*For anyone who has been abused or suffered any other trauma. Objective is to leave the past behind and to think/plan for the future*
41 Loss and bereavement	*Discussion about different types of losses and bereavement to precede the following two scripts, which help deal with any losses or memories that have been triggered by the pregnancy. Addresses having and keeping secrets (e.g. having had an abortion; given a baby up for adoption)*

(Continued)

42 The angels' archway	*For communication with people who have passed over. To be used with clients who believe something exists after living on earth. To help specifically with bereavement and facilitate the grieving process (e.g. death/loss of a particular person; miscarriage or stillbirth). Can be used to work on regrets (e.g. things that were never said or need to be said now)*
43 Letting go of baby	*To work with mums who are not going to keep their baby because s/he will be taken into care; put up for adoption; brought up by another family member; the baby will be given to intended parents by a surrogate*
44 The emotional flowerpot	*For mum or dad who finds it difficult to express their emotions verbally. To enable a client to explore and acknowledge their true feelings about a person or situation. To develop feelings (e.g. of confidence). To promote wellbeing which can be monitored in future sessions by returning to the flowerpot in the greenhouse*
45 Superwoman	*Aims to build confidence by focussing on positive role models/good influences. To develop self-belief and particular skills to help with pregnancy and birthing*
46 The rocky mountain	*Promoting determination to succeed through pregnancy and giving birth. Embedding the idea of being on the right path, being able to deal with any obstacles which are put in the way and being able to change direction at any time*
47 You can so do this	*Promoting self-belief when there is doubt (e.g. not capable of being a good parent; not being able to cope with birthing or caring for a new baby). Specifically useful for young girls and group work*
48 The ballerina	*Metaphor for confidence and achievement. Especially effective for women who have been abused, bullied or have little support. Imagery is included for stretching and remaining focussed during birthing*
49 Sadie	*Metaphor for very young mums who have experienced poor parenting, rejection, neglect or abuse. Demonstrates how trust can be built and skills developed in order to provide for a baby*
50 Well done you	*For use in the final session with mum to congratulate and commend her*

Note

1 Mongan, M. (2016) *Hypnobirthing the Mongan Method: the breakthrough approach to safer, easier, comfortable birthing.* 4th edition. London: Souvenir Press.

3 The importance of assessment and evaluation

It is usually a pregnant mum (rather than dad) who rings me up to enquire about attending a pregnancy and birthing group or having some individual sessions; and in some cases, it could be another professional on behalf of mum, such as, teacher, social worker, support worker or nurse. I usually have quite an in-depth chat on this first occasion because I want to explain about:

- Hypnosis: what it is and what it is not
- My own particular way of working
- Using hypnosis for pregnancy and birthing
- What I can offer (group and individual sessions)
- Consent and confidentiality
- Notes and record keeping.

This chat helps me to find out more about mum, her situation and what she wants and needs, and allows mum to ask as many questions as she likes. I sometimes talk to dad (or the potential birthing partner) as well if s/he is around at the time. It is important for people to think about the conversation we have had before committing to anything. It can be helpful for them to speak to other people who might be running pregnancy and birthing groups or hypnotherapists who specialise in working with pregnancy and birthing. They usually come back with more questions, which is a good thing. It is so important to find the right group or hypnotherapist for mum (and dad/ birthing partner).

If someone wants to attend a group, I then send them an assessment questionnaire (see Appendix 3.1). At that time, I also send them a copy of my consent form for information; as I will have discussed consent and confidentiality (see Appendix 3.2). If I have any further questions or concerns after reading the completed questionnaire, I have another conversation with mum (and dad/birthing partner if appropriate). If mum (and dad/birthing partner) are going to have individual sessions then, as with any other client, I will undertake a full assessment in the first session, which can take anything from 30 to 45 minutes (this is free of charge, which is how I practise with other clients) and I then suggest a package. I use the term 'package' rather than the usual 'treatment plan' for pregnancy and childbirth clients. If they do wish to continue, I discuss consent and confidentiality again and get both mum and dad to sign consent forms. I get them to sign separate consent forms because both of them will be going into trance during the sessions (whether it be an individual or group session).

DOI: 10.4324/9781003173779-3

A hypnotherapist will usually have their own standard consent form, which can be used (or refer to Appendix 3.2).

Whether assessing for group or individual sessions, any assessment should be aiming to get information about the following subjects – some of which will not be relevant to all clients but still have to be checked out:

- Personal details
- Contact details
- Significant people in personal/work life: family, friends, colleagues
- Any professionals/workers involved
- Physical health: current and past
- Mental health: current and past
- Medication/treatment/surgery
- Pregnancy: current and previous (if applicable)
- Planned birthing partner (if any)
- Any current issues/problems
- Counselling/therapy: current and/or previous
- Hypnosis: knowledge/understanding/previous experience
- Fears/phobias
- Hobbies/interests
- Reason for attending/objectives/wishes.

Undertaking a proper assessment is vital before working with anyone either in a group or in an individual session.[1] As well as obtaining information from mum and dad/birthing partner, in some cases it can be important to obtain information from other people (with consent). There will be particular situations where other professionals or workers are involved with mum and have a lot of useful information. For example, if a group is going to be run in a school or college, it can be really useful to speak with the teaching or support staff. A social worker may be working a young person (mum or dad) who is in care. It can be useful to have some background information regarding:

- Family/friends/other significant people
- Significant events: recent and past
- Physical health
- Mental health
- Current situation
- Any behaviour problems
- Any risk factors.

Professionals are always concerned about sharing information (and quite rightly so) but as discussed in the next chapter, if running a group, it is important to undertake risk assessments for the safety of the hypnotherapist and for the group members. When running individual sessions, it can be equally important to undertake a risk assessment and get information from other professionals and workers. In some ways it is easier to share information when working with children (under 18 years of age) if it can be argued one is acting in the best interests of the child under the *Children Act 1989*. It is more difficult when working with adults when professionals must be aware of the *Human Rights Act 1998* and the fact that one needs consent from the adult to share information.

Throughout the book I shall keep referring back to the importance of undertaking a proper assessment before commencing hypnosis/hypnotherapy with a client.

Evaluation

Evaluation of practice is extremely important no matter how experienced a hypnotherapist may be. As professionals and practitioners, none of us ever stops learning. It is vital for all of us to reflect on our practice and learn from it (our successes and our mistakes – because we all make them, e.g. things we wish we had never said or regret that we had not phrased in a better way). So, to get feedback from clients is important. Student hypnotherapists are encouraged to do this when they are training – as the theory and their learning are put into practice. Good training schools will encourage students to continue reflecting on their practice once they are qualified (and a supervisor should help with this) and this can be done by asking a client to complete a formal evaluation once the hypnotherapy sessions and treatment plan have come to an end.

Evaluations can be undertaken in all sorts of different ways – verbal and written; the latter being the most effective way of obtaining evidence for supervision sessions or Continued Professional Development (CPD) purposes. The hypnotherapist needs to ask him/herself what they want to know exactly from the client and the best way to get that feedback – without making it an onerous task for the client. Questions can be general or very specific and the hypnotherapist can choose to use any of the following types of questions:

- Open: which gives the client freedom to expand
- Closed: yes or no answers
- With gradings: 1 to 10 (1 not good/low; 10 excellent/high) OR with options:
  Very useful [ ] Useful [ ] Not very useful [ ] Not at all useful [ ]
  Very satisfied [ ] Satisfied [ ] Not very satisfied [ ] Not at all satisfied [ ]

The hypnotherapist may already have developed a standard evaluation form which they use for all their clients and this can be used (or amended slightly) for mum or a couple having individual sessions for pregnancy and birthing. If running a group, a specific form may need to be developed; again, this is all dependent on what the hypnotherapist wants to get feedback on exactly, that is, their practice or other things as well. So, some topics an evaluation form might cover are:

- Original objectives/learning outcomes: whether achieved
- Practice: methods, techniques
- Benefits gained
- What was useful/not useful; whether anything could have been done differently
- Other needs
- Information sheets, handouts
- CDs/tracks
- Time of classes
- Frequency/duration
- Venue
- Refreshments (if provided).

When I run a group, I ask for verbal evaluations at the end of each session, but at the end of the final session I give out an evaluation form to complete. However, sometimes people are too tired to write an evaluation there and then and it can be better to send out evaluation forms by e-mail a week or so after the last session. There are pros and cons for both methods. People can forget or are too busy to complete them. The hypnotherapist can choose to leave a longer gap (e.g. a month) before sending out an evaluation form or even wait until after the baby is born.

The hypnotherapist needs to make it clear why s/he is asking for feedback and what s/he is going to do with the feedback received. An evaluation serves a different purpose to a review. However, I have known some professionals use comments from evaluation forms to advertise. The hypnotherapist needs to be upfront and honest and not use any feedback without permission. Some professional bodies do not encourage putting reviews on websites, but if a hypnotherapist does choose to do this then the client has to be named and consent must be gained to do this to be compliant with the *Data Protection Act 2018* and the *General Data Protection Regulation (GDPR) 2018*.[2]

Appendix 3.1: Assessment questionnaire for a pregnancy and birthing group

STRICTLY CONFIDENTIAL

Assessment questionnaire for a pregnancy and birthing group

Please answer the following questions as fully as you can.
   Name of Mum:
   Date of birth:
   Address:
   Telephone/mobile:
   E-mail address:
   Children (if any) – include names and ages:
   Name and address of GP:
   Other significant professionals involved in your care/pregnancy:
   How many weeks pregnant now:
   Due date:

   Name of birthing partner(s) (if applicable):
   Date of birth:
   Relationship to Mum:
   Address:
   Telephone/mobile:
   E-mail address:
   Children (if any) – include names and ages:

1. What are your main reasons for wanting to attend a pregnancy and birthing group?

2. Have you seen a hypnotherapist before? (If yes, how was that experience? Was anything particularly helpful or unhelpful?)

3. How much do you know about hypnosis?

4. What do you know about birthing *(or hypnobirthing)*?

5. If you already have children, please give any details about your experience of past pregnancies/births.

6. How would you describe your general state of health?

7. Do you have any diagnosed medical conditions? (If yes, please give details.)

8. Do you ever experience any breathing difficulties e.g. asthma, hay fever? (If yes, do you use an inhaler?)

9. Have you ever had an operation? (If yes, please state when and what for.)

10. Are you taking any medication? (If yes, please give details.)

11. Have you ever been referred to a psychiatrist? (If yes, for what reason?)

12. Have you any fears or phobias?

13. What are your interests/hobbies?

14. How do you currently relax?

15. Do you have any particular worries about your pregnancy or the birth?

16. Is there any other information you think might be helpful to know before the group sessions start?

Form completed by:
  Date:
  Time:

Appendix 3.2: Example of a standard consent form

Consent to treatment, confidentiality and information sharing

I declare that I understand and agree with the following statements:

- I shall engage in hypnosis/receive hypnotherapy treatment from *(name of hypnotherapist)*.
- The limits of confidentiality have been explained to me and I have had the opportunity to discuss this and to ask any questions about things I do not understand.
- On some occasions, sessions may be audio-recorded; this will not happen unless I agree.

- Everything discussed in hypnosis/hypnotherapy sessions or information given in other ways (e.g. telephone, written documents, e-mails, text messages) will remain confidential to *(name of hypnotherapist)* unless a concern arises about: (i) a client who may harm him/herself or another person; (ii) a child who may be at risk of harm/abuse or (iii) there are legal reasons which necessitate the sharing of information.
- Where someone is at risk of harm/abuse this information may be shared with others on a 'need to know' basis (e.g. acting under the *Children Act 1989/2004*; the *Crime and Disorder Act 1998*; the *Domestic Violence, Crime and Victims Act 2004*).
- Written notes will be taken by *(name of hypnotherapist)* during sessions and will be stored safely in the office(s) of *(name and address of hypnotherapist)*.
- Records are also kept in electronic files in the office(s) of *(name and address of hypnotherapist)*.
- All records (written and electronic) will be stored safely and kept in accordance with requirements stated under the *Data Protection Act 2018* and the General Data Protection Regulation (from 25 May 2018), the retention period being up to [X] years.
- *(Name of hypnotherapist)* can contact me by:
  Telephone [ ] Text [ ] E-mail [ ] Letter [ ]

Name of client:
Date of birth:
Address:
E-mail address:
Signature:
Witnessed by *(signature of hypnotherapist)*:
Date:
Time:

Notes

1 I am talking here about assessment in general, but want to highlight the fact that currently with the ongoing pandemic a hypnotherapist is required to undertake a Covid-19 risk assessment the day before working with a client face-to-face.
2 Anyone not familiar with the new data protection requirements should refer to the Information Commissioner's Office: https://ico.org.uk/

4 Running a group

There are numerous hypnobirthing groups and classes available and many are offering similar things. I have already expressed my concern earlier that some people running such groups or classes may not be properly qualified. I believe that in order to run any sort of group work in a professional capacity you need to have undertaken some form of specialist training or gained experience from observing an expert at work. Anyone who has attended any sort of group (whether it be a professional working group, social group, book club, political group or sports club) knows that when you bring a group of individuals together there is going to be a lot of group dynamics going on. Even when you are there for the same purpose or you think you are with like-minded people, conflict can affect the interaction. As a facilitator or group leader you need to know how to handle people firmly, fairly and sensitively and to be prepared for a variety of situations which may arise.

I felt it was important to discuss in-depth the practicalities of setting up and running a pregnancy and birthing group because I do not think it is given enough (if any) attention in books concerned with hypnobirthing. In my career as both a social worker and a hypnotherapist I have run all sorts of groups (e.g. carers' support groups; groups for children on orders/in care; groups for children/adults who have been abused; exam anxiety groups; relaxation groups, to name but a few) and even now I never stop learning and hopefully am always improving my practice. Group work requires developing skills, which will improve through experience (good and bad). It is not something you can just decide to do on a whim. I want to discuss below some important aspects of and considerations for setting up and running a group for mums and birthing partners. Some of the questions posed to the hypnotherapist will also be relevant when planning individual sessions.

I use the term pregnancy and birthing group because I think a hypnotherapist needs to decide what type of group they are going to run, which will be discussed below. Suffice to say, some hypnotherapists may want to run groups which are totally focussed on teaching hypnobirthing, that is, the theory, language, a particular method and techniques. Other hypnotherapists may want their groups to learn a variety of methods and techniques, which offer a broader perspective and alternatives.

I know that some hypnotherapists work remotely and may choose to run classes for pregnancy and birthing this way. The discussions which follow are based on running face-to-face sessions, but the questions raised will also be relevant to sessions run remotely.

Things to consider and plan for

Some of the things I am going to discuss below are a bit like a chicken and egg scenario – what should come first? The answer is you should do what you feel most comfortable

DOI: 10.4324/9781003173779-4

with – especially if you are a newly qualified hypnotherapist or new to hypnobirthing or inexperienced in running a group. The subjects I discuss below are not presented in any particular order of importance – they are all important.

Potential members of a group

Who am I running the group for?

This may seem like a strange question to start with because some might think the answer is obvious – pregnant women or pregnant couples. Part of my reasoning for writing this book is to encourage hypnotherapists not to run stereotypical hypnobirthing groups but rather to think outside of the box. This will become clearer as the discussion progresses below. The hypnotherapist may want to run groups for different target groups – for example:

- Mums who are going to be in a one-parent situation
- Couples only (and maybe specific types of couple)
- Dads only
- Young girls (below 16 or 18 years of age); pupils or students in school/college
- Women who have been raped/sexually abused/force married/trafficked
- Surrogates and intended parents.

Hypnotherapists should consider the possibility of running groups solely for dads or birthing partners too; remembering that this could include all sorts of people. Just one example being, that there could be a pregnant dad, that is, a transgender person who has not fully transitioned. I do want to emphasise the fact that there will be women who will choose to attend on their own; or they have no choice because of their circumstances (e.g. partner works away; partner is in prison). The hypnotherapist can choose to work with couples only or to run a group specifically for single/one-parent mums. Having a mix is good but it is important not to make assumptions and sensitivity is needed in advertising so a mum is not put off by the prospect of being surrounded by stereotypical happy, pregnant couples. From the outset, the hypnotherapist needs to be thinking about how they are going to market and advertise the groups in order to attract the client group with whom they want to work.

Teaching and topics to be covered in a group

Once the hypnotherapist has decided what sort of group s/he is going to run, the content of the classes needs to be considered and a programme developed.

What am I going to cover in the classes?
How will I teach/present the information?

The hypnotherapist needs to plan for:

- Subject areas to be covered
- Methods of teaching
- How information will be presented

- Techniques to be taught
- Exercises
- Structure/agenda for each class
- Information sheets/handouts
- Providing CDs/tracks for practice
- Selecting appropriate music.

If a hypnotherapist has been taught a particular method of hypnobirthing (Leclaire, Mongan or KGH[1]) then s/he will have been given a suggested programme to work to and of course this can be adapted. Some Continued Professional Development (CPD) courses (face-to-face and online) provide ready-made PowerPoint presentations and handouts. For someone newly qualified this might seem like a good safety option until more confidence is developed through practice and experience. Other hypnotherapists might feel they want to be more creative and develop their own programme, teaching style, presentations and techniques.

Whatever the hypnotherapist decides to do, s/he needs to allow enough time to prepare and develop resources. Thought must be given to costs, for example, if information sheets and handouts are going to be given to members of a group; and whether they will be provided in paper format or sent electronically. If CDs/tracks are going to be provided, it takes time to make these and again there can be a cost implication. The hypnotherapist needs to find suitable music and maybe pay for a licence. There are a lot of things to plan for but it is essential to decide what is going to be covered in the classes. Some possible topics which may be included are:

- Hypnosis: what it is; how it can help; the benefits
- Self-hypnosis
- Relaxation
- The body and mind in pregnancy: promoting wellbeing
- Stages of pregnancy
- Stages of labour
- The process of birthing
- Dealing with the unexpected
- Health issues: diet; exercise
- Particular issues in pregnancy, e.g. morning sickness; high blood pressure
- Breathing exercises
- Learning the techniques
- Preparing for the birthing
- Bonding with baby.

Size of a group

Having decided what topics are going to be covered in the group classes, another question needs to be asked:

How many people do I want to work with in a group?

As I have already said it is important for the hypnotherapist to feel comfortable, not just the potential clients. A newly qualified hypnotherapist or someone who is new to working with pregnancy and birthing groups might want to work with a smaller group of people at first. Another consideration is that some potential clients might be put off if they think it is going to be a large group. Some people would never even consider attending a group in the first place. So just to repeat another point I have made elsewhere about marketing – in any adverts it is important to stress the maximum size of a group. As an alternative for those who do not like groups, the hypnotherapist may offer individual sessions, so if this is the case it should be made very clear.

Some mums will want to come to a group with someone else (not dad) and again the hypnotherapist needs to give this some thought. Many mums will attend with a potential birthing partner, which could include a wide range of people so a couple could comprise of:

- Male/female
- Lesbian/gay/non-binary
- Pregnant daughter and mum (in-law)
- Pregnant woman and friend
- Pregnant woman and professional.

Thought must also be given to the possibility that a couple might want to attend with a surrogate. Consequently, there could be a trio attending, but another possibility is a quartet. This can happen when the preferred birthing partner has a job that takes them away frequently or unexpectedly and a 'reserve' birthing partner needs to attend the group. There is potential for a group to be much larger than originally planned for and hence another reason why an initial assessment on the phone (followed up by a questionnaire) is absolutely essential. In any marketing material, it is important to use clear and factual terminology. For example, it is not helpful to say '3 couples maximum in each group'. Some potential clients might immediately feel excluded, for example, a single mum, a gay couple with surrogate or a quartet as discussed above.

Venue

Where am I going to run a group?

Depending on who the group is being run for, a group could run in a variety of locations. For example:

- Hypnotherapist's normal practice location
- School/college/university
- Residential/communal setting (e.g. children's home; prison)
- GP's surgery.

Hypnotherapists can work in a variety of practice locations; some prefer to work from home, so that leads to the question:

Do I have enough room to run a group in my house?

If running a group from home it is important to think about privacy and confidentiality; especially if a group is going to run at a weekend or in the evening when other members of the household might be at home.

Other therapists have their own therapy rooms or they hire therapy rooms; a similar question arises:

Is my therapy room big enough to run a group?

This leads to:

Do I need to hire a venue?

If a hypnotherapist is going to hire a venue specifically to run a group then s/he needs to decide what they want from a venue as well as a number of other things before going to look at actual venues:

What do I need in a venue?
How much do I want to pay?

Some very basic things to consider before going to look at venues are:

- Location: how easy it is to get to by car; whether it is on a bus route; whether it is considered to be a safe area
- Parking: car park; street parking; metered parking
- Disabled access
- Room size
- Toilets
- Kitchen
- Privacy: whether other people will be using the building at the same time the group is running. This is an important factor for maintaining confidentiality.
- Noise: inside and outside the building (case example: church hall was hired. The hypnotherapist had not been told that bell-ringing practice would be happening on that particular night of the week – starting half an hour after the class had begun).

Room and equipment

Looking at venues is a bit like viewing houses to buy; instead of feeling the 'wow factor' it needs to feel right for a pregnancy and birthing class – so it's the 'ambience factor'. The hypnotherapist also needs to think about what equipment might be needed, what is available in the venue and what they might provide themselves.

What equipment might I need?
What equipment can the venue provide?
What am I going to provide myself?

Possible equipment which might be needed:

- Chairs
- Tables
- Mats
- Pillows/cushions
- Blankets/fleeces

- Whiteboard (if giving any presentations);
- Flipchart stand and paper
- Laptop
- CD/DVD player.

Refreshments

Will refreshments be needed/provided?

What might be needed will be dependent on the duration of the classes as some hypnotherapists choose to run half or full day sessions rather than shorter 1.5 or 2 hour classes. A decision needs to be made about what the hypnotherapist is going to provide or whether group members will be asked to bring their own refreshments. We all have our own way of working. I personally always provide bottled water for all my clients no matter whether I am doing group work or individual sessions.

Day and time

I think deciding when to run a group is one of the most difficult decisions the hypnotherapist has to make. The bottom line is you cannot get it right for everybody. If a number of classes can be offered on different days that is the ideal but usually very unrealistic. Some mums (and birthing partners) will be working during the day and will prefer evening or weekend classes. Others who work night-shifts may prefer a class in the day. Therefore, it is more or less impossible to answer the question:

When is the best time to run a class?

There is really no typical working day anymore. Years ago, for office-based workers it was thought to be 09.00 to 17.00. Nowadays people do work more flexible and sometimes very long hours. A lot of people commute every day and cannot get to a class which starts early in the evening. As mum progresses through her pregnancy, she may get very tired and want to go to bed early. The hypnotherapist may try to work around group members if they can be flexible; other hypnotherapists may have to work around their own long-term commitments. Mum is obviously very important, but the hypnotherapist needs to think about him/herself as well:

What time of day do I function best?
What other regular work/personal commitments or clients/family/friends might I have to work around?

The hypnotherapist must think about their own wellbeing too; not just the wellbeing of their clients. Running groups can be both physically and emotionally draining.

Frequency and duration

Another major consideration is:

How many classes should I run?
How long should the classes run for?

The number of classes will be dependent on what the hypnotherapist wants to cover, that is, what subject areas and how they are going to teach (this is discussed further below). Some hypnotherapists choose to run a group over full or half days split over separate weekends. I personally prefer not to run groups like this as I think learning techniques gradually over a period of weeks is more beneficial. Members of the group can go away and practise what they have learnt (over a week or fortnight) and then come back and discuss how things have been for them. If groups run over a number of weeks then members are not only learning and practising, but also building up support networks at the same time. My own preference is to run group classes for two hours. When checking out venues, the hypnotherapist should be mindful that some venues will not charge for setting up and clearing away times (usually allowing 15 minutes at each end of the hours booked). However, some venues will charge for the extra time; it is important to allow for this when calculating costs.

Fees and deposits

All the discussion above leads to the question:

> *How much am I going to charge?*

This is the million-dollar question and I know a lot of hypnotherapists dither or ago-nise over this – especially if they are newly qualified or do not have much experience in working with pregnancy and birthing. Some hypnotherapists will just charge their normal hourly rate times however many hours the classes amount to, or if running a class over a weekend, their normal half or full day rate. The fee would be the same for an individual mum or couple (and yes that might seem unfair and hypnotherapists can decide *not* to do that and offer an individual mum a lower rate). Realistically, potential members of a group need to feel they are getting some sort of bargain or discount, so very often a package will be offered at a reduced price and the adverts emphasise what is included – particularly any extras, such as book; CD/track; information sheets. If a trio or quartet is going to attend (and therefore take up places in the room), the hypno-therapist might want to think about a different fee for them.

It is advisable to take a deposit when someone is accepted into a group, that is, after an assessment has taken place and they want to book a place, which leads to more questions:

> *How much deposit will I take?*
> *When will balances be paid?*

A decision needs to be made about when balances should be paid by. It is better to obtain the balance before a group starts rather than take payment on the day/night, because people can get ill, change their minds. If they pay up front you know they are serious.

> *How will I accept payment?*

There are many options for the hypnotherapist:

- Cash
- Cheque

- Online bank transfer
- PayPal
- Debit/credit card (there are many good, affordable card machines nowadays, e.g. SumUp, Zettle, Square).

All hypnotherapists should have a cancellation policy in place, but it is worth mentioning here that terms and conditions regarding failure to take up a place in a group should be stated clearly on any adverts and explained verbally when talking about fees initially.

Cost should not be a prohibitive factor

For a long time, ante-natal classes were free through the National Health Service (NHS). Nowadays, they are few and far between. The National Childbirth Trust (NCT) offers groups but there is a cost. Private practitioners offer hypnobirthing and again there is a cost. Not everyone can afford to pay for hypnotherapy or go to a pregnancy and birthing group class. Therefore, hypnosis or hypnobirthing is not easily accessible for everyone. Poverty is still a huge issue in our society and certainly is not given enough attention. Pregnancy and birthing group classes and hypnotherapy sessions are not cheap. However, some hypnotherapists (including myself) may offer to reduce their fees or work pro-bono when a client is unemployed, on minimum wage or experiencing financial difficulties. Hypnotherapists may also go to work in schools and colleges, where funding can be secured (e.g. pupil premium; or through an education trust) enabling young girls to access the help and support they need. Hypnotherapy should not be for the elite but it is often perceived this way by others, evoking images of 'yummy mummies' from the middle or well-off classes.

Having a baby can be costly and in our very materialistic society today there is great emphasis through advertising on having all the right things for the baby. It is useful to remember that women have been giving birth for thousands of years in all sorts of places; and although mortality rates were higher, many babies survived with minimal resources and gadgets. Pregnancy and birthing groups can be good as support networks for women (and men) but sometimes the inequality and competitiveness that develops within them is very damaging.

Advertising

Advertising has been mentioned in the discussion above but I wanted to reiterate that the hypnotherapist needs to be careful when advertising their pregnancy and birthing services. Not everyone is going to be in a happy relationship – if they are in a relationship at all. The choice of words and images needs to be given a lot of thought; sensitivity is of paramount importance. I think a key marketing point to make is regarding the benefits of using a properly trained, qualified and registered hypnotherapist. This needs to be stressed on all advertising materials:

- Leaflets/postcards
- Website
- Social media
- Community forums.

Screening

It is possible to see via the internet that many hypnobirthing groups are advertised and potential clients can sign up online and then they just turn up for the class. As stated previously, I think this is very dangerous practice indeed. The hypnotherapist should undertake a thorough assessment in order to screen potential members of a group. This is for the safety of the hypnotherapist and the group members. My practice is to undertake an initial assessment by having a telephone conversation (this could be up to 30 minutes) and then I send out a questionnaire for completion (see Chapter 3).

It can be important to obtain information from other people (with mum's consent) in certain circumstances, such as, other professionals/workers who are involved with mum. For example, it might be necessary to get more information about mum's health from a GP, but sometimes mum might be vulnerable or certain things might have happened in the past which it would be helpful for the hypnotherapist to know about (e.g. from a social worker or teacher), which leads us to think about safety issues.

Health and safety/lone working

The screening process will be the start of a risk assessment process in order to ensure the health and safety of the hypnotherapist and group members. It is important for the hypnotherapist to know who they have got in the group – whether there are any health issues or potential for violence or aggression. This can be incredibly difficult to assess. If a group is being run in a school, a college or perhaps a residential setting, other professionals may have the necessary information regarding risk factors and triggers in order to predict the potential for violence. It can be useful to obtain information about:

- Current problems
- Social history
- Past incidents
- Behaviour (triggers)
- Mum's potential for violence
- Other people's potential for violence, e.g. ex-partner; family/other members of the community of a forced married victim
- Previous losses/bereavement: talking about these issues could upset some group members.

The hypnotherapist running a group could find themselves on their own before or after a class has taken place. They will probably be alone when travelling to and from a venue. In the following chapter, I raise the issue of lone working for hypnotherapists who intend to do home visits to pregnant clients and include some advice regarding what should be included in a risk assessment and an action plan. The discussion is also relevant for any hypnotherapist who runs a group, because at times they will be alone and could be vulnerable.

So, there is an awful lot of thinking and planning to be done before starting a pregnancy and birthing group, and lots of other questions might come into the hypnotherapist's mind (in either the conscious state or trance state!) but for ease and a starting point Appendix 4.1 summarises the key questions which have been discussed in this chapter.

Appendix 4.1: Summary of essential questions

Who am I running the group for?
What am I going to cover in the classes?
How will I teach/present the information?
How many people do I want to work with in a group?
Where am I going to run a group?
Do I have enough room to run a group in my house?
Is my therapy room big enough to run a group?
Do I need to hire a venue?
What do I need in a venue?
How much do I want to pay?
What equipment might I need?
What equipment can the venue provide?
What am I going to provide myself?
Will refreshments be needed/provided?
When is the best time to run a class?
What time of day do I function best?
What other regular work/personal commitments or clients/family/friends might I have to work around?
How many classes should I run?
How long should the classes run for?
How much am I going to charge?
How much deposit will I take?
When will balances be paid?
How will I accept payment?

Note

1 See: https://www.leclairemethod.com/; https://us.hypnobirthing.com/; https://www.kghypnobirthing.com/

5 Individual sessions

Not everyone is a group-type person, that is to say, not everyone enjoys being part of a group, group discussions or having to socialise with other people. This could be for any number of reasons – a person may be shy or simply very private (that is, they do not like anyone knowing their personal situation, thoughts, feelings etc); or they may be suffering with general or social anxiety. Therefore, a pregnancy and birthing group would not be for this type of person. Individual sessions would suit them much better; and in fact, in my own experience a lot of people actually prefer to have individual sessions rather than attend a group. When I use the term individual, I mean a face-to-face therapy session and this could be with a couple, that is, mum and birthing partner or even a trio (surrogate and the intended parents). The main benefit is that the hypnotherapist can design a specific package for mum on her own; or mum and a birthing partner; that is, it is tailor-made. A lot more specific work can be undertaken and there can be more flexibility regarding planning and timetabling of sessions.

When running individual sessions to help with pregnancy and birthing, the hypnotherapist will probably function and work as they normally do in their day-to-day practice. There are certain issues I wish to discuss specifically in relation to this area of work, but if the reader has skipped the previous chapter because they have no intention of running a group, I would suggest you do read it as some (not all) of the questions raised and topics discussed will be relevant to individual sessions.

Most of the basic topics included in group classes would still be covered in individual sessions, but some could be excluded depending on mum's knowledge and experience. Some pregnant women spend hours and hours Googling about pregnancy and know so much already that it really is not necessary to allocate a lot of time to health and education. Also, if mum has children already she may not need to know about the stages of pregnancy/birthing, but will have come for hypnotherapy for a reason or need specific to her. Below is a reminder from the previous chapter of some general topics which might be included when working with someone in relation to pregnancy and birthing:

- Hypnosis: what it is; how it can help; the benefits
- Self-hypnosis
- Relaxation
- The body and mind in pregnancy: promoting wellbeing
- Stages of pregnancy
- Stages of labour
- The process of birthing

DOI: 10.4324/9781003173779-5

- Dealing with the unexpected
- Health issues: diet; exercise
- Particular issues in pregnancy, e.g. morning sickness; high blood pressure
- Breathing exercises
- Learning the techniques
- Preparing for the birthing
- Bonding with baby.

Things to consider and plan for

The hypnotherapist who is going to provide sessions to help with pregnancy and birthing will probably work in very much the same way s/he does with other clients and will not have to plan in the same way they might do for a pregnancy and birthing group as discussed in the previous chapter. Nevertheless, it is worthwhile mentioning a few things here. Just to reiterate, when I talk about an individual session, I mean one which could be for:

- Mum
- A couple (i.e. mum and a birthing partner whoever that may be)
- Surrogate mum and intended parents.

As stated in Chapter 3, it is acceptable to do a preliminary assessment and use questionnaires when thinking about putting a pregnancy and birthing group together. However, when the intention is to work with a mum/couple/trio having individual sessions then it is imperative to do a thorough assessment in order to come up with 'a package' as I call it rather than a treatment plan, which I use in my normal practice with clients.

Hypnotherapists do vary in the way they undertake assessments in their day-to-day practice. Some are happy to do a detailed assessment over the phone or to send a potential client a questionnaire, which has to be returned before the client attends for an appointment. Others (like myself) will have a fairly detailed chat on the phone, but I always emphasise that a proper, full assessment will be undertaken in the first face-to-face session if they decide to book an appointment. An assessment usually takes between 30 and 45 minutes, but in complex cases it has taken me up to an hour. Subjects which are covered in an assessment with any client will be:

- Basic details
- Significant people
- Physical health
- Mental health
- History of treatment/surgery (if any)
- Current medication (if any)
- Experience of therapy/counselling (if any)
- Fears/phobias
- Full discussion of presenting issue/reason for attending
- Interests/hobbies/leisure
- Objectives/goals.

Having done the assessment, it should be possible for the hypnotherapist to discuss possible options for a package. I always emphasise when chatting on the phone that I do not charge for the assessment and if they wish to proceed when the assessment has been completed then we shall carry on for another hour or hour and a half (which is chargeable).

What I like about designing individual packages for pregnancy and birthing is the opportunity to be really creative. Let us take the simple example of a couple coming for their first session. The pregnancy has come as a surprise and they have very little knowledge about pregnancy and birthing. They believed they would be thinking about children much later on in their adult lives. Education is going to be an essential topic to include in the package (in contrast to a mum who has had two babies previously and is unlikely to need the education aspect of pregnancy to be included in her package). It comes to light in the assessment that dad cannot stand the sight of blood. He panics if he does have to look at any type of injury; he cannot watch any hospital documentaries on the television; he has always hated visiting hospital wards in case he sees anyone being given blood through a drip. Part of the package is to book in a separate one-to-one session for dad to work on his phobia (in some cases this might need more than one session). Therefore, a package can include sessions for a couple together or one-to-one sessions for individuals. Another example, might be that a surrogate has some concerns which stem from some of her past personal experiences, but she does not want to discuss this in front of the intended parents. A surrogate could also develop concerns through the pregnancy about her feelings in relation to giving up the baby; that is, she suddenly realises she is going to find it more difficult than she had anticipated when she took on the role (a script is presented in Chapter 43 to help with this).

In my own practice I specialise in working with adults and children who have been abused. There may be issues which mum wants to talk about and work on but her partner has no idea about the history of abuse. Similarly, dad could have issues related to his past that he does not want mum to know about. I feel that most issues which come to light (often mid-package rather than during the initial assessment) do so because of:

• Low self-esteem
• Self-doubt
• Lack of confidence.

The hypnotherapist is likely to deal with such issues in the same way as they would in normal practice but will work on a one-to-one basis with mum or dad/birthing partner. I think it might be helpful to students and newly qualified hypnotherapists to be aware of some typical issues which might be presented:

• Worried that s/he will not love the baby
• Being convinced that s/he will be a bad parent
• S/he had a bad parent and assumes s/he will also be a bad parent (thinking it is hereditary)
• Does not know/understand what good parenting skills are.

So how many sessions?

Again, I have to make the point that hypnotherapists work in different ways and this is in regard to length of sessions too. Many hypnotherapists run their sessions (for adults) for 50 minutes or up to an hour. Others (like myself) prefer to work in longer sessions, unless the client has a particular difficulty regarding concentration span (e.g. an adult with learning disabilities). I usually run my sessions for 75 or 90 minutes. With my pregnancy and birthing clients, I usually book them in for 90 minutes, but have been known to increase this to 2 hours for some couples. Usually, three sessions will be sufficient to cover the basics. Where there are other presenting issues then the number of sessions will be discussed with mum and dad/birthing partner and it can be suggested that extra sessions are included in the package.

Home visits

Mention also needs to be made regarding the location of sessions. Some hypnotherapists will not entertain the idea of doing home visits at all and that is their choice. I do home visits and that probably emanates from my social work background and the fact I have been used to working that way for decades. Some couples do prefer to have individual sessions at home, so it is worth considering whether this service can be offered.

Health and safety/lone working issues were discussed in the previous chapter in relation to running a group, but it is important to raise them again and in more detail for the hypnotherapist who is going to offer home visits. The hypnotherapist must undertake a proper risk assessment and also develop an action plan in order to minimise the risk of harm occurring. Both the risk assessment and action plan should be written documents. I would suggest that if the hypnotherapist has not attended a 'lone working' training course or webinar they should do so as soon as possible.

A risk assessment needs to consider and record:

- Risk-taking action (i.e. doing the home visit)
- Benefits (to the hypnotherapist and client)
- Hazards (anything that could stop the benefits or cause the dangers)
- Dangers (the worst feared outcome, i.e. physical or mental harms).

In order to prevent the dangers occurring, an action plan needs to be developed showing that the hypnotherapist has put some preventative measures in place, for example:

- Mobile phone
- Tracking system
- Personal alarm
- Buddy system.

A buddy might be a family member, friend, colleague or supervisor, who needs to know the following regarding the hypnotherapist and their proposed home visit:

- Location
- Expected duration of visit/appointment
- Mobile number
- Car registration (or bus/taxi firm to be used)
- Who to contact in an emergency
- Agreed 'reporting in' time
- Agreed action if the 'reporting in' time is missed.

Fees

The hypnotherapist who delivers individual sessions for pregnancy and birthing will normally charge their hourly rate pro rata. I am always very conscious of the fact that not everyone is financially well off; and I believe that therapy should be accessible to as many people as possible. Through financial constraints some couples may to prefer have shorter sessions and spread them out over a longer period of time. If the hypnotherapist is going to do home visits, s/he needs to factor into the fee travel costs and the time spent travelling. It is up to the individual hypnotherapist to decide how far they want to travel or whether they prefer to stay local.

Part II

Getting into trance and relaxation

6 The rainbow scarf

Introduction

The main objective in using this script in a first class/session is to introduce the client(s) to trance and achieve deep relaxation. It can be used with just mum, both mum and dad/birthing partner or in a group. It is really important in any first session to get mum (and anyone else attending) relaxed. A client may be very nervous for a whole variety of reasons so, after building rapport and undertaking an assessment, the hypnotherapist needs to introduce them to trance and start to teach them to relax. This script facilitates relaxation but also offers a way that a client can practice self-hypnosis, that is, a gentle way of getting into a deeper trance state. It focuses on the colours of the rainbow, so it is not advisable to use it with someone who may be colour blind (even though in the trance state they may not be colour blind, they could be anxious about this condition and it can be best to avoid it in this initial session).

The script

I want you to imagine that you are outside taking a nice gentle walk. It is a pleasantly warm day. The sun is out and shining brightly, but not too brightly. You are feeling comfortable and well – looking forward to taking a walk in the park which you know is just a short distance away.

You are getting close to the park now. You can see some railings and a pathway that leads into the park. Carry on walking into the park. Take a deep breath in and enjoy the fresh, clean air you are taking in *(and giving to your baby)*. Now breathe gently out. It feels so good. Keep breathing nice and steadily as you continue to walk forward.

Breathe in – and breathe out – that's right. Keep walking forward. I wonder what you are seeing around you. Maybe some other pathways – grass – soil – shrubs – bushes – flowers – trees. I wonder if there is any wildlife about. Maybe birds – squirrels – rabbits – even a hedgehog perhaps. I wonder if you can hear anything. The sound of people chatting together. Children playing and laughing. Birds singing. Bees or wasps buzzing.

As you continue to walk forward you see in the distance a very large tree. It has a wide, sturdy trunk and the tree is also very tall. As you are looking at the tree you notice something tied around the trunk. You can't quite see what it is but you do see a wide band of different colours: violet – indigo – blue – green – yellow – orange – and red.

You keep walking forward towards the tree – fascinated by the different colours. You are drawn towards the tree – curious to see what is tied around it. As you get closer you feel more and more relaxed with each step that you take. Becoming more and more

DOI: 10.4324/9781003173779-6

relaxed. Look at the colours: violet – indigo – blue – green – yellow – orange – and red. It is a very strange thing but as you look at the colours you feel a soothing sensation moving from the top of your head, down through your body and into your feet as they take you towards the tree.

You are nearly there now and as you draw closer you see that it is a beautiful silk scarf that is tied around the trunk of the tree. Go closer now – right up to the tree. Touch the silk scarf – feel how soft and smooth it is. Look at the colours again: violet – indigo – blue – green – yellow – orange – and red. You suddenly come to realise that these are the seven colours of a rainbow: violet – indigo – blue – green – yellow – orange – and red.

Now you will notice that there is a knot tied in the scarf – holding it securely in place around the trunk of the tree. Untie the knot gently and slowly. When you have done that start to unravel the scarf from the trunk of the tree. Walk around the tree to unravel the scarf. Just imagine the tree trunk relaxing as the scarf is unravelled – the whole tree is relaxing – from the very top – down to its deepest roots. All its branches just relax and become floppy. Keep unravelling the rainbow scarf. The more you un-ravel the scarf, the more you feel relaxed. The more the tree is relaxing too. Unravelling the scarf is relaxing you and soothing you. Becoming more and more relaxed. Keep unravelling.

As you keep walking around the tree unravelling the rainbow scarf, you realise that it is a very long scarf indeed. There seems to be no end to it – just like there seems no end to the feeling of being completely relaxed and soothed. Now keep hold of the scarf and gently pull it with you as you start to walk away from the tree. There is no end to the rainbow scarf. You can walk as far away from the tree as you like. There is no end to this wonderful feeling of being relaxed and soothed.

Keep walking until you find somewhere to sit down – somewhere where you can feel really comfortable. Maybe you want sit on the grass; or maybe you prefer to find a seat or a bench. Just find somewhere where you feel really comfortable. Just nod your head when you have found the right place for you to sit or lie down – where you can feel really comfortable.

Hold the rainbow scarf in your hands. Feel how soft and smooth the silk is. Now you are going to focus your attention on each individual colour – one at a time. In a mo-ment I shall begin to count down from *7* to *1*. When I mention a colour look deep into it and see all the different shades of dark and light. The deeper you look into a colour, the deeper you will go into a relaxed state. So now take a deep breath:

7: Look at the beautiful rich violet colour. Look deep into it and relax more deeply
6: Go to indigo – looking into the colour and as you do so you are going deeper and deeper
5: Blue – feeling more and more relaxed
4: Green – as you continue to relax more and more, you feel calm and comfortable
3: Yellow – letting go of everything – any cares or worries – feeling perfectly safe as you go deeper and deeper
2: Orange – even more relaxed now. Feel that wonderful sense of true, deep relaxation
1: Red – as deep as you want to go. Perfectly relaxed, calm, comfortable and safe.

(Guidance note: at this stage if you are working with mum alone you can ask her:

Look at the colours and tell me which one you find most relaxing

If you are working with both mum and dad/birthing partner or a group then say:

Look at the colours again and remember which one you find most relaxing

You can discuss which colours they chose and anchored when they are back in the conscious state)

Now look at the colour you find most relaxing. Look deep into it and as you are doing that enjoy the feeling of true relaxation and hold the rainbow scarf really tight in one of your hands. Look at the hand that is holding the rainbow scarf. You can experience this wonderful feeling of true relaxation at any time in the future – wherever you may be – even with your eyes open. All you have to do is imagine you are holding the rainbow scarf in your hand and say silently or out loud the colour which you find most relaxing. At other times, you might want to take your time to get into this deep state of relaxation, so all you have to do is walk into the park and find the big tree with the rainbow scarf tied around its trunk. Then slowly unravel the scarf and walk away from the tree.

7 The hypno mat

Introduction

Hypnotherapists are always suggesting to clients that their imagination can take them anywhere they want to go and achieve anything they really want to do. The hypno mat is useful in demonstrating the power of the imagination in a first session either with an individual (not just mum) or in a group. A key message is that going into trance and distracting oneself can help with so many issues. Travelling on the hypno mat demonstrates this in a fun way by showing how one can take control and go anywhere. The hypno mat can also be used to go somewhere to create a safe place or it can be the safe place. If the client likes the hypno mat it can become a place to practise in the future – relaxation, distraction and other techniques which are learnt. Finally, the script can also be used in conjunction with scripts from Part X for ego boosting because it promotes looking after oneself and there is a great emphasis on wellbeing.

The script

Your subconscious mind is a very powerful thing. It is a reliable friend – always there to help and protect you. It will help you achieve anything you really want to do. Your subconscious mind is there to help you work on any issues or problems you may have, but it is also there to help you with your wellbeing – both your physical and mental health.

It is all too easy in this fast society we live in to neglect yourself and your wellbeing. In your life you probably play a lot of different roles and have a range of responsibilities. Maybe you sometimes put other people and their needs before yourself and your needs. Caring about or for others is a wonderful quality to have but you still need to look after yourself on a daily basis. It is important to make time for yourself every single day. You are important. Promoting your wellbeing and looking after yourself is essential. Don't fall into the trap of using that old cliché: 'I'm too busy'. You need to make time for yourself. Going into trance every day and using self-hypnosis is a good way to relax, to feel good and maintain your physical and mental health in order to promote your own wellbeing *(and the wellbeing of your baby)*.

Your subconscious mind can take you to any place you want to go in your imagination. You can go to places you know and like; you can visit your memories. Or you can just let your subconscious mind take you anywhere it wants to go – on a magical mystery tour – that can be really exciting. What is important is that you take time out to relax every day and have time for you.

DOI: 10.4324/9781003173779-7

Now in your imagination you can travel anyway you want – use any mode of transport. What you might find useful though is to use your very own hypno mat. It's a bit like a magic carpet. It can take you anywhere. So just imagine what your hypno mat might look like. Just imagine it now. I wonder what it looks like.

(Guidance note: what follows are some prompts the hypnotherapist might use if required)

What shape is it?
What colour is it?
Touch your hypno mat.
What is it made of?
How does it feel?

When you are ready, I want you to either sit or lie down on your hypno mat. Do whatever is most comfortable for you. As you get comfortable on your hypno mat, you feel as though you are sinking into more comfort – a deeper sense of relaxation. Comfort and relaxation. Just sink down – that's good. Enjoying comfort and relaxation. As you are enjoying this wonderful feeling of comfort and relaxation, I want to say a few things to you. As you become more relaxed my voice might drift in and out – and you may miss some of what I say – but that really does not matter at all.

As you are resting comfortably there on your hypno mat remember that you are important. Your wellbeing is important. It is not selfish to think that you are important. You are important to you. You are important to others too. That is why you need to take care of yourself and take positive actions to promote your wellbeing every day of your life.

(Guidance note: if working with mum(s) only insert the following:
Inside your body you are carrying a baby, who is relying on you now and will continue to rely on you for a long time into the future – as s/he grows from being a baby into a toddler – into a child – into an adolescent and finally into an adult. So, you need to look after yourself – keep well physically and emotionally for you and your baby)

It is important to keep fit and well. Feel satisfied. Feel joy. Feel happy. Have a positive approach to life – not letting stress or worries *(if working with an individual insert anything else that is specifically a negative for that person)* hinder you or hold you back in any way. Think positive thoughts and use positive language always.

Remember too that you can always take control. You can change any thought, feeling or behaviour if you really want to do so. You are in control of your hypno mat. You can use it any time you like in the conscious state or in trance state. All you have to do to summon it is to say to yourself either silently or out loud: 'hypno mat'.

It is so comfortable and relaxing lying on your hypno mat, but remember your hypno mat can take you on lots of different journeys. It might be fun to take a journey now. On the count of *3* your hypno mat will start to move – *1, 2*, and *3*. Off it goes. Remember you are in control. You can tell your hypno mat what you want it to do. So have a bit of fun experimenting with it now.

Tell it to go faster. Now tell it to slow down. Choose which direction you want it to go. I wonder if you will choose right, left, up or down. I wonder what else your hypno mat can do – swerve – turnover – spin – take a leap.

(Guidance note: if working with an individual the hypnotherapist can ask what is happening – where s/he is going and will then follow as s/he goes on a journey.)

If working with mum, the hypnotherapist can use this opportunity to gain more information for assessment, that is, whether mum is visual, auditory, kinaes-thetic, olfactory or gustatory. Some standard prompts/questions [which can be explored further, and obviously dependent on where mum goes] follow)

Where are you now?
Do you see anything?
What do you see?
Is anyone there?
Do you see any wildlife?
Do you sense anything around you?
Do you hear anything?
Do you smell anything?
Do you taste anything in your mouth?
Can you touch anything which is nearby?
How is the temperature?
Do you want to change anything?
How are you feeling?

Now I want you to tell the hypno mat to find somewhere very safe for you – a place where you can return to at any time when you are in trance and also when you are in the conscious state. A place where you can feel calm and at peace.

(Guidance note: a safe place can then be created using the hypno mat to find it and then it should be anchored. Alternatively, the hypno mat can become the safe place)

Well, that was fun wasn't it? You can have fun any time you want on your hypno mat. Go anywhere you want in your imagination. It is also there for when you want to prac-tise self-hypnosis and practise the things you are going to learn to help you *(and your baby through your pregnancy and birthing)*. All you have to do is say to yourself either silently or out loud 'hypno mat'.

8 Marshmallows

Introduction

This is a very simple script to help introduce mum to trance but it can also be used as a deepener. Its primary objective is to get her to relax and it is a good script for mum to use and practise self-hypnosis herself after the first session. Some mums who really like the giant marshmallow use it as a safe place. Please note that mums who have been told that they are having a boy or girl may see their giant marshmallow as blue or pink – and that is absolutely fine. Some hypnotherapists may prefer to ask whether the giant marshmallow mum is seeing is white, pink, blue or any other colour.

The script

Just close your eyes and make yourself as comfortable as you can. Have a wriggle about if you need to – so that your body is feeling in a good, supported position. It is time for you to experience some relaxation and learn how to go into a deep trance state. It is good to have a variety of ways of doing this and it is also good for you to practise going into trance at least once a day so that you get some relaxation regularly – when nothing else and no-one else intrudes.

Let your mind drift. It does not matter where it goes. Your mind is free to go anywhere it wants to go. Just think about having some time for yourself. This is a time to relax and not to think about anything in particular. Just let your mind drift naturally and easily.

When you need to relax it is good to have a place where you can go in your mind and get comfortable. Very much like you are doing now. I just want you to imagine that you are standing somewhere – it does not matter where – and in front of you, you see a giant marshmallow. It is absolutely huge – much, much bigger even than a king-size bed. I wonder what colour it is. It looks so soft and inviting. It would be lovely to go and lie on it.

Walk towards the giant marshmallow and stop when you are right next to it. Just put your hand on the marshmallow and feel how soft and squelchy it is. Push your hand down on the marshmallow. As you do that you will experience a strange sensation – a rush of lightness will go down your whole body. Do it again – push down on the giant marshmallow – feel that rush of lightness again in your own body. And again – push down on the giant marshmallow – feel that rush of lightness again in your own body. Such lightness.

DOI: 10.4324/9781003173779-8

The giant marshmallow is so soft that you might like to lie on it. Climb onto the giant marshmallow and then lie on your back. You feel your whole body – from the top of your head to the tips of toes – sinking down into the giant marshmallow. Sinking down – experiencing a wonderful sense of relaxation. The whole of your body – inside and out – is just relaxing and becoming floppy. Just as your mind is relaxing more and more you feel that sensation again through your whole body – lightness – but now you also feel support and safety. Lightness – support and safety – whilst lying on the giant marshmallow.

As you sink further down into the giant marshmallow look up to the ceiling above you and you will see ten smaller marshmallows on the ceiling. You realise that a stream of light is coming out of each individual marshmallow – streaming down onto the giant marshmallow. These ten marshmallows are going to help you go into a deeper relaxed state. In a few moments I am going to count from *10* down to *1,* and when you hear me say a number the light from one of the marshmallows will be switched off and you will sink into an even more relaxed state. You will feel as though you are sinking deeper and deeper into the giant marshmallow. So now...

10: The light from one of the marshmallows goes off and you relax even more

9: Another light goes out. You are letting go of everything in your mind

8: Any cares or worries you have been carrying in your mind just leave you now

7: Your whole body is relaxing slowly and gently

6: Any aches or pains you may have been experiencing recently leave your body now

5: Half the marshmallow lights have gone out now. Double your sense of relaxation

4: Feeling lightness – supported – and safe

3: Double your sense of relaxation now

2: Feeling deeply relaxed – not a care in the world

1: You are feeling totally relaxed – lightness – supported and safe.

(Guidance note: the hypnotherapist can then decide where they want to take mum having got her into a deep trance state)

9   Counting watermelon seeds

Introduction

This is another simple script to get mum, dad/birthing partner or a group into the trance state by visualising and counting.

The script

Just close your eyes and start breathing nice and slowly. Breathe in – *1, 2, 3* – and hold. Now breathe out slowly – *3, 2, 1* – relax. That's good – now try that again. Breathe in – *1, 2, 3* – and hold. Now breathe out slowly – *3, 2, 1* – relax. Now just keep breathing nice and slowly – feel more relaxed and calmer with each breath that you take. As you keep breathing nice and slowly you are beginning to feel more and more relaxed.

Now just imagine that you are holding one of your arms straight out in front of you – with the palm of your hand facing upwards. In the palm of your hand, you are holding a watermelon. Just look at the watermelon in your hand. Focus your attention and look at the outside of the melon. Look deep into the green colours you see. Look at the patterns on the skin. Maybe you see some lines or mottled shapes. With your other hand feel the outside of the watermelon. Feel how smooth it is to touch.

I wonder how much the watermelon weighs and whether it feels light or heavy in the palm of your hand. Maybe your hand is starting to feel heavy with holding the watermelon. Maybe you feel your arm getting heavier and heavier. As it is getting heavier and heavier this might be a good time to see inside the watermelon.

So, imagine that you are carrying the watermelon to a table where you see a knife and a spoon. Pick up the knife and slice the watermelon in half – then lay out the two halves. Look at one half of the watermelon. Look at the flesh of the watermelon – I wonder whether it seems pink or more like red to you. Look deep into the flesh and see the different shades of pink or red. I wonder if you can see any patterns within the pink or red flesh. Now turn your attention to the other half of the watermelon. Look at the flesh – look deep into the flesh and see the different shades of pink or red. I wonder if you can see any patterns within the pink or red flesh.

Now look at both halves of the watermelon again. Focus your attention on the black seeds within both halves of the watermelon. Now an interesting fact you may or may not know about a watermelon is that a watermelon can have anything between 200 and 800 seeds inside of it. That is a lot of seeds for one watermelon. Just look at the black seeds in the two halves of the watermelon. I wonder how many seeds your watermelon has got.

DOI: 10.4324/9781003173779-9

Focus your attention now on just one half of the watermelon. Look at the black seeds. I wonder if you might try to guess how many black seeds might be in that half of the watermelon. Just think of a number in your mind. Now take the spoon from the table and start spooning out the black seeds – just one at a time. As you place a seed on the table start counting back from whatever number you thought of – now spoon out another seed and count backwards. Keep spooning out the seeds – one by one – keep counting backwards. As you are spooning out the seeds you feel more and more relaxed – spooning down and down into the flesh of the watermelon. With each number you count – you feel more and more relaxed. Keep counting backwards – going deeper into the flesh of the watermelon – feeling more and more relaxed.

Part III
Breathing

10 Breathing

One of the most important things a hypnotherapist should do with any client is to talk about breathing. Most of my clients look at me with a quizzical look on their face when I say: 'I'm going to teach you how to breathe'. I then go on to explain what I mean and why practising breathing on a regular basis is so important for everyone (not just pregnant women!).

Life in general is very fast nowadays. Technology has developed so quickly to enable us to have more of ways of communicating. Very often the expectation is that someone should be available 24/7 and respond immediately to any communication received whether it be an e-mail, text message or voicemail. Such expectations and way of life put people under immense pressure and are the reasons why stress levels can go through the roof. A lot of human beings put others before themselves. Clients often tell me they feel guilty taking time for themselves. When life is busy and time is tight it is easy to neglect oneself. Being busy and spending life in a hurry affects one's breathing; and often this lifestyle results in a person finding it hard to relax.

I believe that teaching breathing exercises and using scripts to help clients slow down their breathing and relax is a vital part of any hypnotherapist's work. It lays the foundation for therapeutic work in future sessions. I usually suggest to clients that they should practise their breathing at least four times a day. For pregnant women learning to breathe in a variety of ways is of paramount importance in order to prepare for birthing.

Some pregnant women will already know how to breathe in a good way because they have taken yoga classes, they meditate or perhaps use mindfulness. Some pregnant women will come to a hypnotherapist because they want to learn hypnobirthing techniques specifically. The hypnotherapist needs to be clear in their marketing literature what they intend to offer, that is, hypnobirthing techniques only or other options. There are different methods of hypnobirthing and the hypnotherapist may choose to follow a particular one or take from the different methods. I think it is very worthwhile if the hypnotherapist can take the opportunity to learn about the main methods (e.g. Leclaire, Mongan or KGH)[1] and if s/he prefers a particular method to undergo specialist training as part of their CPD.

When teaching general breathing techniques, the hypnotherapist will often follow the structure:

Say: Breathe in
Count: *1, 2,* and *3*
Say: Hold
Say: Breathe out

DOI: 10.4324/9781003173779-10

Count: *3, 2,* and *1*
Say: Relax.

The client is learning how to breathe slowly but also learning how to control the air they take in and then let out. I think this is a good starting point when working with a pregnant woman too, but in later sessions it is important to teach other types of breathing for the birthing, that is, the breathing needs to be continuous – not holding at any point.

No matter what the reason is for a client seeking some help from the hypnotherapist, all hypnotherapy should be client-led. What I mean by that is, the hypnotherapist in the initial assessment must find out as much as possible about the client in order to decide the best way of working with them, that is, what will be suitable techniques, which will then be incorporated into a treatment plan. When a pregnant woman wants to use hypnosis to help her through her pregnancy and the birthing process, I think it is very important to assess what is going to work best for her and I then develop what I call a 'package', rather than a treatment plan.

Teaching breathing exercises as part of the package should be fun and not seen as a test or a chore. There are many different techniques – not all of them will suit a client – most clients will have their favourite(s). It is important to find out what suits the client best in regard to counting, which will be discussed further below.

Breathing and hypnobirthing

Hypnobirthing has developed over many decades now and the main advocates have developed their own methods and techniques. For example, Marie Mongan[2] suggests that there are three gentle breathing techniques in Hypno-Birthing:

* Calm (for relaxation between contractions)
* Surge (for when contractions have started – when the cervix is opening and thinning)
* Birth (for breathing the baby down).[3]

Whereas Katharine Graves[4] focusses her work on:

* Up breathing (for the first stage of labour)
* Down breathing (for when the baby is moving down the birth canal).[5]

The hypnotherapist who is running a pregnancy and birthing group has less time to experiment with a group than the hypnotherapist who is providing individual sessions. If time allows, I think it is best practice to go through as many breathing techniques as possible and mum will decide which ones help her best and she feels most comfortable with.

Counting

The hypnotherapist will usually start to teach breathing using number counting. A well-trained hypnotherapist will have learnt about the speed of counting and practised relentlessly to develop their skills in order to get it right. Some people struggle to breathe in for a long count. Some of the techniques Mongan teaches include counts of

8 and *20*. Some of my clients have struggled with a count of *5* or *6*, so it is important to adapt and work with what suits the client best.

There are so many different ways the hypnotherapist can teach breathing techniques and they may be called by different names. However, most of them could be broken down into three types of breathing exercises known as:

- Number
- Ratio
- Colour.

So, whether I am running a pregnancy and birthing group or providing individual sessions, I go back to basics because I believe this is a good starting point. When I teach the hypnobirthing techniques, I always explain that these are specific to hypnobirthing and in my own practice I do take from the different models mentioned above.

Number breathing

Number breathing involves breathing in for a certain number count and then breathing out for the same count. The main objective is to slow the breathing down and be able to control it – especially when breathing out. I usually start with a count of *3* and explain that eventually (after a week) this can be increased – firstly to *4* and then after another week to *5*.

> Breathe in: *1, 2, 3* – and hold
> Breathe out: *3, 2, 1* – relax.
> Breathe in: *1, 2, 3, 4* – and hold
> Breathe out: *4, 3, 2, 1* – relax.
> Breathe in: *1, 2, 3, 4, 5* – and hold
> Breathe out: *5, 4, 3, 2, 1* – relax.

Ratio breathing

This type of breathing requires more control. It involves breathing in for a certain number count and then taking double the time to breathe out. Some clients can struggle with this at first. It is good to start with *2* and *4* and gradually increase to *3* and *6*. On occasions I have had clients that build up to *4* and *8*.

> Breathe in: *1* and *2*
> Breathe out: *4, 3, 2,* and *1*
>
> Breathe in: *1, 2,* and *3*
> Breathe out: *6, 5, 4, 3, 2,* and *1*
>
> Breathe in: *1, 2, 3,* and *4*
> Breathe out: *8, 7, 6, 5, 4, 3, 2,* and *1*.

Colour breathing

It is important to ascertain what is the negative colour and what is the positive colour for a client. This can be undertaken in a variety of ways, depending what the issue is.

This technique is used a lot for people who suffer with anxiety or experience panic attacks, but I have found it also works well for mums in the birthing process. Colour breathing has two stages. So, I shall use a very simple generic example which might be used when a client is fearful.

Stage 1

I just want you to breathe in slowly for *3* and then gently breathe out for *3*.
Breathe in – *1, 2, 3* – and hold. Breathe out – *3, 2, 1* – relax.
That's good and again.
Breathe in – *1, 2, 3* – and hold. Breathe out – *3, 2, 1* – relax.
Now you just keep breathing at your own pace. Whilst you are doing that, I want you to remember the last time you felt *(fear or insert another negative emotion)*. Just keep breathing slowly. Now think about that last time. Think about where you were – what you were doing. Keep breathing.
Breathe in – *1, 2, 3* – and hold. Breathe out – *3, 2, 1* – relax.
Continue to think about *(fear/other negative emotion)* and remember how you were feeling. Stay with that feeling.
Breathe in – *1, 2, 3* – and hold. Breathe out – *3, 2, 1* – stay with that feeling.
Breathe in – *1, 2, 3* – now see a colour.

The hypnotherapist then asks the client what colour s/he saw. This will be the negative colour. The hypnotherapist will then explain the technique. Instead of thinking about the last negative experience, the client focusses on the colour. Each time the client breathes out the colour will start to fade. The client is encouraged to breathe out (or even blow) hard. The client continues breathing until the colour fades completely.

Stage 2

I just want you to breathe in slowly for *3* and then gently breathe out for *3*.
Breathe in – *1, 2, 3* – and hold. Breathe out – *3, 2, 1* – relax.
That's good and again.
Breathe in – *1, 2, 3* – and hold. Breathe out – *3, 2, 1* – relax.
Now you just keep breathing at your own pace. Whilst you are doing that, I want you to remember the last time you felt really happy or go back to a memory you have where you were so happy.
Just keep breathing slowly. Now think about that happy time. Think about where you were – what you were doing. Keep breathing.
Breathe in – *1, 2, 3* – and hold. Breathe out – *3, 2, 1* – relax.
Continue to think about being happy and remember how you were feeling. Stay with that happy feeling.
Breathe in – *1, 2, 3* – and hold. Breathe out – *3, 2, 1* – stay with that happy feeling.
Breathe in – *1, 2, 3* and see a different colour now.

The hypnotherapist then asks the client what colour s/he saw. This will be the positive colour. The hypnotherapist will then explain the second stage of this technique. The client will focus on the positive colour and start breathing it in.

Now focus on that beautiful positive colour.
Breathe in – *1, 2, 3* – and hold. Breathe out – *3, 2, 1* – relax.

Look deep into the *(colour)*. Look closely – look at the different shades of *(colour)*. I wonder as you look more closely whether you see any patterns or shapes within the *(colour)*.

This beautiful *(colour)* is full of relaxation and calmness. As you take a deep breath in you will feel the relaxation and calmness and it will start to move around your body. The relaxation and calmness will relax every part of you inside and out. Just feel everything relaxing – becoming calmer – inside and out.

Take another deep breath and breathe in the *(colour)* – *1, 2, 3* – and as you breathe slowly out feel the relaxation and calmness travelling all around you – inside and out.

As you continue breathing in and out, you will continue to feel more relaxed and calmer.

Breathe in – *1, 2, 3*. Now breathe out – *3, 2, 1*. Relaxed and calm.

What follows

The discussion above has focussed on the importance of teaching general breathing exercises for any client, but these exercises can be a good starting point for a pregnant client too. Mum should learn these techniques and then progress to learn specific techniques for the birthing process. I think it is imperative that any dad or birthing partner should be involved in learning the techniques too; they should be fully participative in any exercises, so they can learn to relax themselves and also support mum.

The following three chapters contain visualisations and scripts which can facilitate the learning of breathing techniques; other techniques are then included in scripts throughout the book.

Notes

1 https://www.leclairemethod.com/; https://us.hypnobirthing.com/; https://www.kghypno birthing.com/.
2 Mongan, M. (2016) *Hypnobirthing the Mongan Method: the breakthrough approach to safer, easier, comfortable birthing.* 4th edition. London: Souvenir Press.
3 Mongan, M. (2016), pp. 151–160.
4 Graves, K. (2017) *The Hypnobirthing Book: An inspirational guide to for a calm, confident, natural birth.* 2nd edition. Marlborough, Wiltshire: Katharine Publishing.
5 Graves, K. (2017), pp. 41–51.

11 Visualisations

Introduction

Using visualisations can be very effective in helping with movement and smooth movement is obviously an essential part of the birthing process. Visualisations facilitate the development of effective breathing and distraction techniques but they can also help with the passing of time. In hypnobirthing there is a lot of discussion and teaching around up and down breathing (attributable to Katharine Graves and the KHG method[1]) and movement of muscles. In some hypnobirthing texts the visualisations are very short (e.g. a couple of sentences) and certainly can serve a useful purpose. However, in my own practice I have written visualisations which are longer and can be used in individual or group sessions. I then encourage mum to decide which she finds most helpful and to start practising every day. This is an ideal opportunity for dad/birthing partner to get involved by reading out the visualisations for mum to practise. I suggest dad/birthing partner types or writes the favoured visualisations on cards (some prefer to use a mobile phone or iPad), which they can use during the birthing, whether it be at home or in hospital. As mum and dad/birthing partner practise together, they amend what is written on the cards; they become a work in progress. When working with a group I will put the visualisations I use in a session into a handout, which can be used at home.

What follows are visualisations which are divided into:

- Up breathing
- Down breathing
- Up and down breathing.

Up breathing is used in stage 1 of labour, that is, when contractions (or waves or surges) are occurring and the muscles of the uterus are being drawn upwards. The breathing technique is:

Breathe in slowly through the nose – then breathe out gently through the mouth.

Down breathing is used in stage 2 of labour, that is, when the cervix is fully dilated and the baby starts his/her journey down the birth canal. The breathing technique is:

Breathe in quickly through the nose – then breathe out slowly through the nose.

Counting can be used whilst visualising but is not always necessary once mum is well-practised in breathing. If counting is used, I explore what mum feels most comfortable with, so she does not feel it is like a test.

DOI: 10.4324/9781003173779-11

Up breathing

1 Bunches of balloons

Hold your hands out in front of you. Now look down at both your hands and realise that in each hand you are holding a bunch of coloured ribbons. Each ribbon is very long. You can see all different colours. Look at one of your hands – it does not matter which one – look at the bottom of the long, coloured ribbons you are holding in your hand and follow the ribbons upwards. You see that each ribbon is attached to a balloon. The balloons are all different colours too. Count how many balloons there are. Now look at your other hand and look at the bottom of the long ribbons and follow the ribbons upwards. You see more balloons. Count how many balloons there are.

Open one of your hands and see all the balloons start to float upwards – going up, up and up. Going higher and higher into the sky. Keep watching the balloons as they keep going up, up and up. Going higher and higher. Dispersing in different directions – travelling so lightly – feeling free – finding their own pathway upwards high into the sky. Now open your other hand and see all the balloons start to float upwards – going up, up and up. Going higher and higher into the sky. Keep watching the balloons as they keep going up, up and up. Going higher and higher. Dispersing in different directions – travelling so lightly – feeling free – finding their own pathway upwards high into the sky.

2 Flying a kite

You are in a huge open space somewhere out in the open. There is no-one around. It is a very windy, blustery day. You are wrapped up warm in a coat, hat, scarf and gloves. It is a really good day for flying a kite. Look at your hand – you are already holding a kite. Look at the body of the kite. You see a frame and outer covering. Look at the shape of the frame – follow the shape. Then look at the outer covering. Notice what the frame is made of and then what the covering is made of. What colours do you see? Is anything drawn or written on the kite? You will also notice the long tail dangling down which will help the kite to fly even better. Take control of the kite now – hold the line. You are in complete control. You can and you will control the movement of the kite in these windy, blustery conditions. When you are ready let the line go – release the kite. Watch the kite start to fly up, up and up. The kite is flying with the wind. See it fly high up, up and up towards the sky. Up and up it goes. Going with the wind – not fighting it just going with it – flying in the wind. Up, up and up. It's going even higher and higher now. Up, up and up.

3 Cable car up the cliffs

You are standing on a beach. When you turn one way you can see the sea. When you turn the other way, you see very high cliffs. They look insurmountable, but it is always possible to find a way up. As you look along the beach you realise that there is a cable car. You see a group of people waiting to get into it. You realise this is how people get up the cliffs very quickly. Walk along the beach now towards the cable car. You see the people getting into the cable car and the doors close very quickly. The cable car starts to move upwards. Just watch it on its journey towards the top of the cliffs – upwards towards the landing. See the cable car climbing up the cliffs – up, up and up it goes.

A quarter of the way up. Now half way up the cliffs. Still travelling up, up and up. Three-quarters of the way up now. Almost there. Up, up and up. Nearly there – almost at the landing. Up, up and up – and then it stops at the landing – it's arrived.

4 Creatures in the sky

You are looking up into the clear blue sky. There are no clouds to be seen anywhere. You see the clear blue sky and the bright yellow sun. Bring your gaze a little lower and start looking for all the different creatures that might be moving upwards in the sky and are trying to reach the sun. Moving up and trying to reach the lovely warm sun. Look for the birds – so many types of birds – maybe sparrows, robins, blue tits, crows, ravens – flying up and up and up. Maybe you hear the sounds of bees buzzing first before you see them flying around but then going up and up and up towards the clear blue sky. Then maybe you hear some wasps before you see them going up and up and up towards the clear blue sky. Now you see some beautiful butterflies. Look at the different colours of their wings. All these creatures are lifting upwards – flying around – going higher and higher – going up and up towards the blue sky and the beautiful yellow warm sun.

5 Butterfly house

You are going to walk around a butterfly house. It is a special visit which has been arranged for you only. No-one else will be there, just you and the butterflies. So, take a deep breath in and walk through the two plastic doors which form the entrance to the butterfly house. As you go through the doors you feel the humid heat hit you like a wave – but you adjust – it may be different from outside where you have just come from but you get used to the heat very quickly. You realise that the heat can actually be very soothing and comforting. You look above you and see a clear glass ceiling that gives a perfect view of the sky. Then looking directly in front, you see lots of greenery – thin bamboo trees – rubber plants – shrubs – plants and beautiful tropical flowers you have never seen before. They look so intriguing you want to take a closer look. There are so many different colours to look at in the tropical flowers. So, you start walking forward – there are several pathways you can take – you choose which way you want to go. As you are walking forward and looking at all the greenery, butterflies start flying around you. Landing on your arms – your shoulders – even on your head. Look at all the different types of butterflies – the different colours on their wings. Keep watching the butterflies – watch how they move – now watch the ones who are flying upwards. Upwards towards the tall trees. Upwards towards the top of the bamboo trees. Upwards towards the glass ceiling. Flying upwards and upwards.

Down breathing

1 Raining round the lake

You are walking around a really big lake that is surrounded by large, tall trees with lots of branches that are covered in green leaves. The place where you are walking feels spacious and safe. Just as you are looking across the lake you realise that it is starting to rain. You keep on walking. The rain continues to fall. Watch the falling rain – look at the droplets falling from the sky – down, down, down and down onto the pathway. You keep walking and watch the falling rain – down, down, down and down. Focus on the rain falling down – it feels soothing and relaxing as you watch the rain fall down, down, down and down. You do not want to shelter from the rain and delay your journey – you want to carry on walking – getting to your destination. Keep looking at the rain – the raindrops falling from the sky – down, down, down and down. Keep going. Keep walking. Watch the rain falling – down, down, down and down. That's right – you are getting there. Keeping going. Keep walking. Keep watching the rain falling – down, down, down and down. By continuing to walk you are reaching the end of your journey.

2 Bouncing ball

You see a staircase that goes from the attic which is in the top of a large, old mansion house right down to the ground floor where the front door leads out of the house. The staircase goes down through several landings. It twists and turns. You are standing at the very top of the staircase and in your hand, you have a bouncing ball. In a moment you are going to bounce the ball on the top step of the staircase and then watch it bounce down, down, down and down – down each individual step – all the way down to the ground floor. You are going to watch the ball bounce down each step of the staircase. Bouncing down, down, down down and down.

Now bounce that ball. Watch it go down, down, down and down – bouncing down each step. Look how high it bounces. It reaches the next landing. Now it starts down the staircase again bouncing down, down, down and down each step. Look how lightly it is bouncing. It reaches the next landing. And again, it starts another part of the staircase – bouncing down, down, down and down each step. It is bouncing so easily. It reaches the next landing. Off it goes again – watch it bouncing down each step – bouncing down, down, down and down each step – and it reaches the next landing. Nearly at the bottom now – the final part of the staircase – bouncing down, down, down and down each step – and the ball reaches the ground floor and rolls towards the front door – ready to go through the door and explore outside.

3 Sledging on the hill

It is winter and the snow has been falling for hours and hours now. Snowflakes falling down and down and down – falling continuously from the dark grey sky. The snow has become very, very deep. All the roads, pavements, rooftops, gardens, hedges and fences are covered in a thick white blanket of snow. It is a really good day for going sledging. Imagine standing at the top of a steep hill with a sledge and in front of you all you see is the white blanket of snow – totally unspoilt. Place the sledge in front of you and then get on it. Hold the reins tight. That's right. In a moment you are going to take the journey down the hill. Ready – steady – off you go. The sledge starts slowly going down the hill. Down it goes – gathering speed gradually – taking a steady, straight course. Down and down and down the sledge goes – never going off course. Faster and faster the sledge goes. Leaving tracks behind as it continues to go down and down and down across the white blanket of snow. Halfway down the hill now – going faster and faster – still on course. Down and down and down the sledge goes – getting towards the bottom. Down and down and down the sledge goes. Nearly there now – at the bottom.

4 Chocolate fountain

You are standing in front of a huge banquet table. It is covered in a beautiful, white linen tablecloth. The only thing on the table – right in the middle – is a big chocolate fountain. Look how tall it stands – count how many tiers it has. Nothing is moving yet. All you see is a thin layer of thick, brown chocolate. Then suddenly the top of the fountain starts to move. You see lashings of chocolate bubbling at the top of the fountain and then the chocolate starts running down all sides of the fountain – across the tiers. Watch the thick, brown chocolate running down the tiers of the fountain. Down, down, down and down on its journey to the bottom of the fountain. See the chocolate running down – some parts pouring very smoothly as the chocolate runs down, down, down and down across the tiers. On other parts of the fountain, you see some little ripples within the chocolate as it runs down, down, down and down on its journey down to the bottom of the fountain. The fountain keeps oozing chocolate out from the top – the chocolate moves down, down, down and down the tiers of the fountain. The fountain continues producing chocolate – and the chocolate keeps moving down on its journey – down, down, down and down to the bottom of the fountain.

5 Deep sea diving

You are sitting on a boat in the middle of the sea. You are going to take a relaxing journey down under the sea. You are going to go deep sea diving. Just check your equipment first – your mask is clean so you can see clearly. Your cylinder tank is full of oxygen and your breathing apparatus is in good working order. You have your compass – you know exactly in which direction you are going. You are ready to go on the dive of a lifetime and explore underneath the sea. Jump into the sea and start to swim under the surface of the water. Now swim deeper. You are swimming down and down through the water – down and down – go deeper. Your arms and legs are feeling strong – making good progress through the water – down and down you go. Breathing deeply – plenty of oxygen coming from the tank. All is well as you continue further down and down deeper into the sea. Look around you – so many different things to see. Look at the creatures that live below the sea – all shapes, colours and sizes – watch how they are moving. Now look at the objects and treasures left behind from years and centuries gone by. Down and down you go – feeling strong as you go down and down towards the sea bed. Making good progress – down and down you go. Look at the beautiful colours all around you – the creatures, the objects – down and down towards the bottom of the sea-bed.

Up and down breathing

1 The escalator

Up

You are in a busy shopping centre. There are lots of people about and you feel that you have had enough and want to get away from the crowds. So, walk away from the people – adults, young people and children. Keep walking until you find an escalator. Stand at the bottom of the escalator and watch it for moment. You notice how it is moving – moving with purpose. It moves very steadily and very smoothly. It is on a continuous, purposeful journey. Look at the escalator going up, up, up and up – ready to take you up and out of this place. The escalator has a job to do; it knows exactly where it is going. Up, up, up and up. Step onto the escalator and start your journey upwards. Travelling up, up, up and up – keep going – up, up, up and up.

Down

You have travelled on the escalator before. You're ready now for your journey down on the escalator to your destination. Stand at the top of the escalator and watch it for a moment. You notice how it is moving – moving with purpose. It moves very steadily and very smoothly. It is on a continuous, purposeful journey. Look at the escalator going down, down, down and down. The escalator has a job to do; it knows where it is going – to your destination. Down, down, down and down. Step onto the escalator and start your journey downwards. Travelling down, down, down and down – keep going – down, down, down and down.

2 The lift

Up

Imagine a really tall building. The biggest sky scraper you have ever seen in your life. Bigger than the Great Pyramids, the Shard, the Empire State building or the Shanghai Tower. Now look at that building and see that it has a glass lift on the outside of it. That is the way to get up to the very top of the building. Walk towards the lift. Get into it and as soon as you are in the lift, the glass doors close automatically and the lift begins to move. It lifts off the ground – moving very quickly but very smoothly. The lift is made of thick safe glass so you can see out into the far distance. Keep looking at everything you can see out there – bridges – buildings – houses – hotels – hospitals – museums – traffic – people – animals – trees. Up and up and up the lift rises so very quickly. Search for things you can see on the ground – look at the things you are leaving behind as you go up, and up and up. Now look upwards – high above you. Going up and up and up towards the top. The lift is moving very quickly and smoothly. Up and up and up it goes – nearly at the top now – and then you are there.

Down

You have been in this glass lift before. It is now time to take a trip down to the ground. Get into the lift and as soon as you are in there, the glass doors close automatically and the lift begins its journey downwards – moving very quickly but very smoothly. Down and down and down it goes. I wonder if you will see the same things as you saw before as you travel downwards. Keep looking at everything you can see out there – bridges – buildings – houses – hotels – hospitals – museums – traffic – people – animals – trees. Down and down and down the lift goes so very quickly. Going down and down and down towards the ground. The lift moves very quickly and smoothly. Down and down and down it goes – nearly at the bottom now – and then you are there.

3 The helicopter

Up

You are standing outside on the top of a building which has a helipad. You see that a helicopter is in position – ready for take-off. You can see the pilot checking all the equipment is in good working order. Look at the helicopter – you can see the rotor mast on the top of the helicopter that holds the main rotor blade. The tail rotor blade is right at the back of the helicopter. You know the engine is in good working order and the tank is full of fuel so the helicopter can go as far as it needs to do. The main rotor blade starts spinning round slowly – round and round – then getting faster and faster. As the rotor blade spins round and round getting faster and faster the helicopter starts to lift up off the helipad. The blades are going faster now and the helicopter lifts up, up and up. It lifts up – off the building – flying up, up and away from the building. Flying up, up and up into the sky. Going on its journey – up, up and up. Watch the helicopter as it continues its journey – up, up and up.

Down

You are standing on the helipad watching for the helicopter to return to the helipad. Keep looking out for it – watch for the helicopter. Watch for the dot in the sky. I wonder which direction it will come in from today. Keep looking. There it is – you see the helicopter. It is on the last stage of its journey. It has started its descent – coming down towards the building and down towards the helipad. Watch the helicopter as it flies down, down and down. Getting closer now. Flying down, down and down towards the building and the helipad. The engine is working well. There is plenty of fuel left in the engine – it could keep going if it needed to do so. Getting closer now. Flying down, down and down towards the building and the helipad. Keep watching the helicopter – the strong rotor blade on top and the tail rotor blade at the back. Flying down, down and down towards the building and the helipad. Getting closer and closer – and then it lands on the helipad.

Note

1 Graves, K. (2017) *The Hypnobirthing Book: An inspirational guide to for a calm, confident, natural birth*. 2nd edition. Marlborough, Wiltshire: Katharine Publishing.

12 Fanning out

Introduction

Two scripts are presented in this chapter to encourage the idea of the cervix opening up for birthing. It is helpful for mum to visualise anything that spreads out, that is, fans out. A peacock's tail and a flamenco dancer's fan are excellent ways of doing this.

The scripts

In today's session I want you to give some thought to when you are going to be in the final stage of birthing – when your baby is on his/her last part of their journey. You know it is important for you to be relaxed and you have been doing really well practising your breathing and preparing the best way you can. You also know that it is important for the muscles of your cervix to be relaxed when the baby is on his/her journey and about to arrive into the world – the cervix needs to be relaxed and open. So, I want you to imagine certain things that might help your cervix relax and open easily – fanning out in a very natural way.

Script 1: The peacock

I want you to imagine you are out in the countryside taking a pleasant walk in the warmth of the afternoon's sunshine. You are surrounded by lovely green fields and hills that stretch far into the distance. You are enjoying the walk looking at all the beautiful and natural things around you.

Just ahead of you on the pathway you see something move from the hedge on the side. You are not quite sure what it is. Then you see it again. It looks like a blue head popping out and then it goes back in. You are curious to see what it is, so you move closer. There it is again – out and then in. Then suddenly you see a beautiful blue head come out followed by the body of a peacock. The peacock struts out and then turns to face you. It stops still and looks you straight in the eye.

The peacock is looking proud and very confident. He holds his head up high. Then he turns around – so you can see just how long his feathers and tail are. Look at the length of him – from the feathers on the top of his head – right down his body – to the tip of his tail.

Look again from the top of his head to the end of his tail and this time notice all the deep rich colours you can see. On his face you may see black, grey and blue. On his

DOI: 10.4324/9781003173779-12

body and tail you may see different shades of blue, green and yellow. Look deep into the rich, beautiful colours.

The peacock is proud and confident. He knows you are looking at him and he wants to show you how beautiful his feathers are. Suddenly, he lifts his tail high – it is like a big long train of feathers – standing high and straight. Then slowly – very slowly and very gently – he opens his tail – and it fans out – to the right and to the left – far and wide. Watch carefully how the tail fans out – slowly and gently – far and wide. Slowly fanning out – taking no effort at all – just a very natural thing to do. Fanning out – far and wide. Look at all those beautiful colours and patterns in the peacock's tail – fanning out so far and wide. Now it has fanned out – stretched as far as it can. The peacock's tail is a beautiful fan.

Script 2: The flamenco dancer's fan

You are out in a tapas restaurant having a meal. Whilst you are eating the entertainment starts. A female flamenco dancer walks into a small area in the centre of the restaurant. Just watch her begin to dance. She is so confident. She knows the steps. She knows how to present herself. Her head, arms, hands, trunk of her body, legs and feet are all so strong and they work so well together. In one of her hands, she is holding a fan, which is closed. She cleverly flicks it open and fans herself whilst continuing to dance. Everything is flowing and working in harmony. Then she flicks the fan shut again. The dancer never hesitates. She knows exactly what she is doing – with her head, arms, hands, trunk of her body, legs and feet. She knows what steps come next and which direction she needs to go in. Everything flows just as it should. Look how confident the dancer looks – head held high – laughing eyes – smiling face. She is happy – enjoying the experience. It is so exciting to watch. The excitement is contagious – you can feel it all around the room.

When the dance comes to an end for some unknown reason the dancer comes to your table and hands you the closed fan she has had in her hand. She indicates she wants you to have it. She puts the fan into your hands and then holds it there securely. You thank her for the fan. Now, as the dancer walks away from the table, just let the sounds of the restaurant drift into the background – the music – people's voices – the clatter of plates, glasses and cutlery. Just let them all drift into the background.

Look at the closed fan you are holding in your hand. Hold it tight. Look at what it is made of. Feel its texture in your hand. What colours do you see? Feel the expectation and excitement – wondering what the fan will look like when it opens out. When you feel ready, start to open the fan – just do that now. Very slowly open the fan out. See how easy it is to open the fan out. As it opens slowly you will start to see things. Look at what you see in the fan – what the fan is revealing as it opens up. Colours – shapes – patterns – I wonder if it is forming a picture. Keep opening the fan slowly. Opening out – very slowly – a picture is emerging – it is becoming clearer. Even clearer now. The fan is now nearly completely open – what do you see? What is in the picture?

(Guidance note: the hypnotherapist can choose to explore what is in the picture and see where it takes mum. Alternatively or in addition, the hypnotherapist can use the additional text below to guide mum to imagine birthing)

Maybe you can see yourself in the birthing room. The dancer's fan opening out slowly is like your muscles relaxing in the birthing room – helping your baby on his/her journey into the world. The muscles relaxing and fanning out – helping the baby to move down and down and down. Imagine the muscles relaxing and fanning out. Look at the picture in the fan:

What do you see?
Who is in the room?
What is happening now?
What happens next?
What are you doing?
How are you feeling?

13 Breathing with the waves

Introduction

This script can be used purely for relaxation and mums really seem to enjoy this. It is a good one to record with some wave-type music in the background for mum to use at home. When I originally wrote the script, my main objective was to teach mum to breathe for the actual birthing. Floating on the waves in the sea is a lovely place to practise breathing and using the waves can successfully embed the idea of continuous movement. This script encourages continuous, smooth breathing. Other types of breathing can be practised and other work can be undertaken whilst breathing and floating on the waves; and it is also a good place to deal with morning sickness. Some people might think the sway of the waves might make mum feel even sicker, but I find that the gentle sway often calms the waves of nausea. So, I have put in an additional script for this.

The script

Imagine that you are walking along a beach that has beautiful golden sand which stretches far into the distance. There is no-one else about. You sense that the sea is nearby and maybe you can hear the waves. The sun is out and shining brightly – high up in the blue sky. The temperature is just as you need it to be – just right for you. Enjoy walking along the beach. Feel the sand very soft under your feet. Walking slowly and steadily. Enjoy the clean air that you breathe in – and then you breathe out. Keep breathing steadily as you walk – breathe in – and breathe out. Slowly and steadily. Enjoying the perfect peace and calmness that surrounds you.

As you walk along the beach notice what is all around you. Then look at the sea – such an inviting blue colour – so very clean and so very clear. You are feeling drawn towards the sea. You look at the gentle waves – going forwards and backwards – forwards and backwards. Very, very gentle. The waves are just moving forwards and backwards – forwards and backwards. Very, very gentle.

It might be really relaxing to lie on top of those waves and move gently with them. The perfect rhythm of the waves will help you breathe naturally – slowly – gently – continuously. So, walk towards the water and then dip one toe in it. Feel the temperature of the water – it is just right for you. Now put your whole foot in and enjoy the feel of the water. Now walk slowly into the sea – feeling your way – keep walking – further in you go.

Feel the water rising up both your legs – from your feet – to your ankles – to your calves – to your knees – to your thighs. Feel the gentle waves splashing against

DOI: 10.4324/9781003173779-13

your body. The water is rising up towards the top half of your body. When you feel you have gone deep enough – to a point where you feel completely safe – turn around and lie on your back. Just float on your back and look up at the sky. I wonder what the sky looks like today. What colour is it? Is it clear or are there some white fluffy clouds? Can you see the sun? Can you see anything else high up in the sky?

As you are floating on your back – relaxing – become aware of the gentle waves around you. As the waves move gently, they help you to relax. Moving forwards and backwards – forwards and backwards. So relaxing. Relaxing your head – and also supporting your head. Relaxing your back – and also supporting your back. Relaxing both your arms – and also supporting both your arms. Relaxing both your legs – and also supporting both your legs. Your whole body is relaxed, well supported as you continue to float with the waves.

Now close your eyes and feel more deeply the gentle waves – beneath you and around you. Now that you are so relaxed this might be a good time to think more about your breathing and to practise your breathing. Let the waves help you breathe and relax. Breathe and relax.

(Guidance note: the hypnotherapist should decide what count to use with the client; and the count can be increased in future sessions. A good starting point is 3; but aiming to work towards 6 – as used below)

I am going to count to *(say what count is going to be used)* whilst you breathe in and breathe out – floating with the waves. When I mention a body part it will relax immediately – you will feel that body part relax completely. Breathing continuously – never stopping for a moment. You are going to relax each part of your body – both inside and out. Starting at the top of your head. When I mention a body part it will relax immediately – you feel that body part relax completely.

Breathe in: *1, 2, 3, 4, 5, 6.* Top of your head. Breathe out: *6, 5, 4, 3, 2, 1.*
Breathe in: *1, 2, 3, 4, 5, 6.* Both of your ears. Breathe out: *6, 5, 4, 3, 2, 1.*
Breathe in: *1, 2, 3, 4, 5, 6.* Forehead. Breathe out: *6, 5, 4, 3, 2, 1.*
Breathe in: *1, 2, 3, 4, 5, 6.* Eyelids. Breathe out: *6, 5, 4, 3, 2, 1.*
Breathe in: *1, 2, 3, 4, 5, 6.* Eye muscles. Breathe out: *6, 5, 4, 3, 2, 1.*
Breathe in: *1, 2, 3, 4, 5, 6.* Nostrils. Breathe out *6, 5, 4, 3, 2, 1.*
Breathe in: *1, 2, 3, 4, 5, 6.* Cheeks. Breathe out: *6, 5, 4, 3, 2, 1.*
Breathe in: *1, 2, 3, 4, 5, 6.* Lips. Breathe out: *6, 5, 4, 3, 2, 1.*
Breathe in: *1, 2, 3, 4, 5, 6.* Teeth. Breathe out: *6, 5, 4, 3, 2, 1.*
Breathe in: *1, 2, 3, 4, 5, 6.* Gums. Breathe out: *6, 5, 4, 3, 2, 1.*
Breathe in: *1, 2, 3, 4, 5, 6.* Jaw. Breathe out: *6, 5, 4, 3, 2, 1.*
Breathe in: *1, 2, 3, 4, 5, 6.* Neck. Breathe out: *6, 5, 4, 3, 2, 1.*
Breathe in: *1, 2, 3, 4, 5, 6.* Throat. Breathe out: *6, 5, 4, 3, 2, 1.*
Breathe in: *1, 2, 3, 4, 5, 6.* Shoulders. Breathe out: *6, 5, 4, 3, 2, 1.*
Breathe in: *1, 2, 3, 4, 5, 6.* Arms. Breathe out: *6, 5, 4, 3, 2, 1.*
Breathe in: *1, 2, 3, 4, 5, 6.* Hands. Breathe out: *6, 5, 4, 3, 2, 1.*
Breathe in: *1, 2, 3, 4, 5, 6.* Fingers/thumbs. Breathe out: *6, 5, 4, 3, 2, 1.*

Keep breathing with the waves. Forwards and backwards. Feel the waves beneath you and around you – helping you to breathe. Breathing continuously – never stopping for a moment. Now start relaxing the middle of your body.

Breathe in: *1, 2, 3, 4, 5, 6*. Chest. Breathe out: *6, 5, 4, 3, 2, 1*.
Breathe in: *1, 2, 3, 4, 5, 6*. Stomach. Breathe out: *6, 5, 4, 3, 2, 1*.
Breathe in: *1, 2, 3, 4, 5, 6*. Spine. Breathe out: *6, 5, 4, 3, 2, 1*.
Breathe in: *1, 2, 3, 4, 5, 6*. Bottom. Breathe out: *6, 5, 4, 3, 2, 1*.

Keep breathing with the waves. Forwards and backwards. Feel the waves beneath you and around you – helping you to breathe. Breathing continuously – never stopping for a moment. Now start relaxing the lower part of your body.

Breathe in: *1, 2, 3, 4, 5, 6*. Legs. Breathe out: *6, 5, 4, 3, 2, 1*.
Breathe in: *1, 2, 3, 4, 5, 6*. Feet. Breathe out: *6, 5, 4, 3, 2, 1*.
Breathe in: *1, 2, 3, 4, 5, 6*. Toes. Breathe out: *6, 5, 4, 3, 2, 1*.

Keep breathing with the waves. Forwards and backwards. Feel the waves beneath you and around you – helping you to breathe. Breathing continuously – never stopping for a moment. Now start relaxing the inside of your body. All those organs that are healthy and working so well to keep you and your baby safe.

Breathe in: *1, 2, 3, 4, 5, 6*. Heart. Breathe out: *6, 5, 4, 3, 2, 1*.
Breathe in: *1, 2, 3, 4, 5, 6*. Liver. Breathe out: *6, 5, 4, 3, 2, 1*.
Breathe in: *1, 2, 3, 4, 5, 6*. Kidneys. Breathe out: *6, 5, 4, 3, 2, 1*.
Breathe in: *1, 2, 3, 4, 5, 6*. Intestine. Breathe out: *6, 5, 4, 3, 2, 1*.
Breathe in: *1, 2, 3, 4, 5, 6*. Bowel. Breathe out: *6, 5, 4, 3, 2, 1*.

And do not forget how important it is for all the muscles in your uterus to relax all through your pregnancy.

Breathe in: *1, 2, 3, 4, 5, 6*. Uterus. Breathe out: *6, 5, 4, 3, 2, 1*.

Now just keep breathing with the waves and let every single muscle that exists in your body relax all at once.

Breathe in: *1, 2, 3, 4, 5, 6*. Muscles. Breathe out: *6, 5, 4, 3, 2, 1*.

Now just keep breathing with the waves and let every single bone and little vertebra that exists in your body relax all at once.

Breathe in: *1, 2, 3, 4, 5, 6*. Bones and vertebrae. Breathe out: *6, 5, 4, 3, 2, 1*.

So now you are completely relaxed breathing with the waves. You can come into the sea at any time and use the waves to help you breathe and relax. I want you to remember that you can use self-hypnosis to relax and practising self-hypnosis every day is very important for both you and your baby. If you are relaxed and calm – your baby is relaxed and calm. So, just walk into the sea until you are deep enough to lie on your back and float with the waves. Practise your breathing by breathing in and counting to yourself, say a part of your body and relax that part before breathing out and counting down.

Additional script 1: Waving goodbye to morning sickness

(Guidance note: before getting mum into trance the hypnotherapist needs to talk about how the morning sickness manifests itself, that is, how it actually affects mum – what are the exact symptoms – so they can be used within the script)

I know you enjoy floating with the waves in the sea. It is just so relaxing – and you have been so good at practising your breathing here. I know recently you have been experiencing some nausea/morning sickness *(insert whichever is appropriate; morning sickness will be used for the rest of the script)*. Floating with the waves could help you get rid of the morning sickness. Whenever you feel sick again, I want you to come into the sea and get yourself settled on the waves as you know how to do. To get there quickly you just have to say 'waves'.

So, imagine that you are floating gently on the waves. You are experiencing the morning sickness. It is so horrible – waiting to be sick. You have told me how you feel *(insert symptoms as discussed)*. Imagine the last time you felt that way. Now let's take each one of those feelings separately and get rid of them. To do this the sea is going to become very calm. As you are floating there now the waves are going forwards and backwards – just as they normally do when you breathe with the waves. Just imagine that the waves start to slow down – they are slowing down further. As you are feeling the waves slow down you are feeling less and less sick. The waves are slowing down further. You are starting to feel less sick but you still need to get rid of *(insert symptoms as discussed)*. So, one at a time throw them in the sea.

(Guidance note: the hypnotherapist then works with mum to throw each symptom/feeling into the sea)

Have you noticed there are no waves left? The sea is completely still and flat. You no longer feel sick. Your stomach and insides are calm – just like the sea. Any time in the future when you feel sick, come into the sea and slow the waves down and throw away all those feelings. You can control the waves – you can get rid of the morning sickness.

14 Going skiing

Introduction

Hypnobirthing involves the concept of a journey, so it can be really useful to have a number of scripts which take mum on a journey. Some mums appreciate having a choice of different journeys which can be used during the birthing. This skiing script works with the idea of travelling up and down during a journey. It can be used as a practice preparation script but it can also be broken into parts to help with the various types of breathing at different stages of the birthing process. The travel up and the travel down parts of the script can be used as stand-alone mini scripts.

This script will appeal to someone who enjoys skiing (this reiterates again why it is so important to undertake a thorough assessment and find out about a mum's interests and hobbies) but of course it can also be used for someone who has never been skiing but would like to try it. The hypnotherapist can promote the idea that mum can learn quickly and be good at something that comes naturally very quickly (like giving birth).

The script

Today you are going to have an experience on some ski-slopes. I just want you to make sure you are properly dressed and kitted out for the experience. I know you like to be prepared in the best way possible. So just imagine what you might like to wear. You will certainly need some warm underneath clothing – maybe some thermals; but you will also need a ski-jacket, ski-pants and maybe a fleece. So, imagine yourself getting ready. Don't forget you will need some socks and ski-boots; and gloves or mittens.

Tell me what you are wearing *(prompt about colour)*.

Tell me how you are looking *(prompt about how her face is looking; the shape of her body; how she is standing; her body language; what her face is showing)*.

Tell me how you are feeling.

Now you need some equipment to make sure you are safe on the ski-slopes and whilst you are skiing. First of all, go and find some sun-cream for your face to protect you from the sun's rays and the glare from the snow, which can be so bright and strong. Maybe some sunglasses and goggles to protect your eyes. You will need your skis and ski poles. What is really vital is a helmet for your head. Do you think you have everything you need? Is there anything else that might be helpful to you? It is so important to be well prepared for an exciting journey.

(Guidance note: the next section can be used as a stand-alone during the first stage of birthing, i.e. the UP stage)

DOI: 10.4324/9781003173779-14

Travelling up

Right so you are ready and prepared. Looking forward to taking your journey on the ski slopes. Look in front of you and you will see a big white mountain covered in snow – stretching very high up. Now I do not know if you are familiar with the different types of ski slopes – some people call them pistes. Ski slopes are made of compacted snow so they feel very solid. You need to choose which type of slope you want to try on this journey:

- A nursery slope is for a beginner
- A green slope is easy and gentle
- A blue slope is still quite easy – it is slightly steeper but not very deep
- A red slope is considered to be intermediate
- A black slope is for the advanced skier.

So, which one will you choose?

Now see if you can find the chair lift, which is going to take you to where you need to be – at the top of the ski-slope. Can you see it? Good. Can you see the chairs travelling up – up and up? Moving with purpose. Moving steadily and gently. Just watch the chairs. Going up – up and up. Now just make your way towards the moving chairs. They make you feel like you want to travel up – up and up. Keep walking – feeling uplifted – knowing what you need to do. Breathing in through your nose and out through your mouth. Keep focusing on the chair lifts going up – up and up. That's right. Breathing in through your nose and out through your mouth. That's very good.

So, now climb into a chair lift. You – baby and *(dad/birthing partner if appropriate)*. Make yourself comfortable. Ready to travel up to the slope. Feeling excited about the journey and reaching your final destination. There is a little jolt and the chair lift starts to move upwards. Now it is moving very gently. Going up – up and up.

Look around you, what do you see?

As you are travelling upwards, what do you see below you?

What have you left behind?

Keep travelling up – up and up. Breathing in through your nose and out through your mouth. Look up and see the mountain of snow – travelling towards your slope. Look up at the beautiful blue sky and see the sun shining so brightly. Such beauty all around you. Feeling lighter as you continue to travel upwards. Feeling fit and energised – ready to ski and finish your journey. Feeling excited. Feeling confident *(insert any other appropriate suggestions at this point)*.

You are almost there now. Nearly at the slope. Still a little further to go – up – up and up. And you are there. So, get off the chair lift and have a look around. Feel the compact snow beneath your boots – solid and firm. Feel that confidence within you – ready for the journey down. Ready to ski down the slope.

(Guidance note: the next section can be used as a stand-alone during the second stage of birthing, that is, the DOWN stage)

Travelling down

Just look all around you – look at the beautiful white blanket of snow. The compact, sturdy snow. This is such a beautiful place to be in. Look at the blue sky and the lovely sunshine. Everything is good in the world – enjoy the beauty, calmness and peace that surrounds you. Now look down the slope. Can you see right to the bottom? Tell me what you see exactly. Can you see anything on the actual slope? What do you see at the bottom – your final destination? Keep looking down the slope and work out which route you want to take.

Before you start skiing down the slope just practise your breathing. Quick breath in through the nose. Longer breath out through the nose. That's right and again. Quick breath in through the nose. Longer breath out through the nose. Good.

OK – you are ready for the final stage of your journey. You are going to ski smoothly down the slope. You and your baby are going to have a smooth journey together – skiing down the slope – in harmony. On the count of *3* start your journey – skiing down the slope – *1, 2,* and *3.* Off you go. Down – down – down. Remember your breathing. Quick breath in through your nose. Longer breath out through your nose. Down – down – down. Quick breath in through your nose. Longer breath out through your nose. Good – you are skiing so well. You have learnt so quickly. You know exactly which way you are going. Down the slope you go. Down – down – down. You are going faster now – gathering speed. Down – down – down. Enjoy the journey down with your baby.

Look to your right and tell me what you see. Down – down – down the slope you go. Quick breath in through your nose. Longer breath out through your nose. You are doing so well skiing – down – down – down – keep going. You have learnt so quickly. Enjoy the journey down with your baby. Now look to your left and tell me what you see. Down – down – down the slope you go. Quick breath in through your nose. Longer breath out through your nose. Just keep going down – down – down. Feel the strength in your legs and arms as you manoeuvre the skis and ski poles. How skilful you are. How in control you are. So confident in what you are doing. Knowing where you are going – how to get to your destination. Knowing exactly which direction you are going – down – down – down. Knowing you are getting to your destination.

Think about how you are feeling as you move down – down – down. Confident. Strong. In control. Excited *(insert anything else which is pertinent to mum).* And you are nearly there now – at the bottom of the slope. You have done it. You have skied all the way down the slope. You have arrived.

15 Flying high in a plane

Introduction

This is another script to work on the concept of a journey. It should not be used with anyone who has a fear of flying.

The script

Just think about how exciting it can be to go to places you have never been before. Meeting new people. Seeing new things. Having new experiences. Never knowing what you are going to experience next, which is so thrilling. You can feel all sorts of emotions when you go travelling.

I want you to imagine now that you are going on a journey to somewhere you have never been before. You are going to be travelling by plane. So, imagine that you are at the airport. You have already checked in your luggage and you are waiting in the departure lounge. *(Dad/birthing partner if appropriate)* is sitting next to you. You are *(both)* feeling calm and relaxed; looking forward to experiencing something new. You can look out through the huge glass windows to all the runways and lots of planes are parked up on the runways. Some planes are taxiing down the runway; others waiting patiently in a queue ready to take off.

You hear your flight being called. So, stand up and make your way to the gate where your plane is waiting. Show your boarding pass and passport. Walk along a passageway, which will take you to a bus. Get on the bus and wait for it to fill up with other passengers. Suddenly the doors close and you are driven to the plane. It is only a very short journey. The bus stops directly at the bottom of the steps that will take you up and into the plane. Get off the bus now and you see ten steps going up to the door of the plane. When you hear me say a number you will take a step up and feel lighter as though you are stretching upwards towards the sky.

1: Take the first step up
2: And take another step
3: Up you go again
4: Getting nearer to the plane
5: Halfway there now
6: Still climbing up
7: Up and up you go
8: Feeling very light

DOI: 10.4324/9781003173779-15

9: Stretching towards the sky

10: And you are at the door which leads into the plane.

The flight attendants are there to greet you at the top of the steps. You find your way to your seat – you know exactly where to go. So, get yourself settled into your seat; make yourself comfortable and ready for the flight. Do not forget to fasten your seat belt. As you watch other passengers taking their seats and the flight attendants helping some passengers put their hand luggage in the locker above the seats – you feel relaxed but also excited about the journey you are about to take.

So, you hear the engines start. The captain comes over the loudspeaker and welcomes you to the flight. Then the flight attendants start to do the health and safety demonstration. The journey is beginning – slowly but surely. You are confident that you are going to enjoy this journey – nothing to worry about at all.

The plane starts to go forward – taxiing along the runway; crossing a junction where two runways meet and then it joins a queue of planes. Waiting patiently – no need to hurry – all will be well – the plane will take off when the time is right. Slowly moving forward in the queue. The plane is at the front of the queue now. It goes forward and turns onto the runway. The engines, which are in perfect working order, get louder and louder and then suddenly the plane starts to move very quickly and it tilts upwards. The plane is off the ground – rising up and up and up into the sky.

(Guidance note: the next section can be used as a stand-alone during the first stage of birthing, that is, the UP stage)

Travelling up

Just sink further into your seat feeling really relaxed as the plane continues to lift higher into the air – rising up and up and up into the sky. Remember your breathing – breathe in through your nose and out through your mouth. Your breathing helps you to relax even more. Breathe in through your nose and out through your mouth. That's right.

Take a look out of the window. Look down at the ground as the plane rises up and up and up into the sky. See the airport you are leaving behind. The houses that look like little squares. The cars and lorries that look like dots on the roads. Getting smaller and smaller as the plane rises so smoothly – up and up and up into the sky.

The plane is passing through lovely white fluffy clouds. Look deep into the clouds and look at the different shades of dark and light – so soothing. Up and up and up – higher and higher – the plane continues its journey smoothly and safely. Knowing which direction to take – knowing what is right.

(Guidance note: the hypnotherapist can take this script further and work on other issues by introducing the concept of in-flight entertainment:

- *Listen to music (for distraction)*
- *Watch a film (for forward pacing)*
- *Use iPad (deleting files – getting rid of things; creating new files; forward pacing)*
- *Read a book (use for regression or forward pacing)*

The next section can be used as a stand-alone during the second stage of birthing, that is, the DOWN stage)

Travelling down

Now it is time for the final part of your journey – the descent. Pack away everything you have been using on the flight – make sure your seat belt is secure. Feel the plane start its descent – going down – down – down and down. Use a different type of breathing now – take a quick breath in through your nose and then let a longer breath out through your nose. That's right. A quick breath in through your nose. A longer breath out through your nose. Good. Keep breathing – as the plane travels down – down – down and down.

The plane continues its journey down. Going down – down – down and down. You are on the final part of your journey – nearly there – feeling excited about experiencing new things. Doing new things with your baby *(and significant others if appropriate)*. Doing things you have never done before. You are feeling confident that you know what is right for you and your baby. You know you have good instincts – you know what is right. You can try things out – experiment – find out what works best for you and your baby. You will choose to do what is right for you and your baby.

Keep breathing – as the plane travels down – down – down and down. Through the clouds – down – down – down and down. Descending further – reaching the end of the journey. Keep breathing – a quick breath in through your nose. A longer breath out through your nose. As the plane travels down – down – down and down – look out through the window. See the houses – the squares becoming larger. The cars and lorries on the roads – no longer dots – getting bigger and bigger. Nearly there now – reaching your destination. It is so exciting. You are preparing to land. You can see the runway outside of the window – it is getting nearer and nearer – the plane is getting lower and lower. Nearly there – the tyres are nearly on the runway – and then the tyres are on the runway and the plane keeps moving forward but slows down – slowing down and down until it stops. You are at the end of your journey. You have arrived.

16 Let's imagine water

Introduction

Water is a very relaxing visualisation which can be used to calm a client, unless of course s/he has a fear or phobia regarding it. Therefore, it is important that the hypnotherapist has checked for any fears and phobias during an initial assessment. The script which follows has a general introduction to get mum into trance and then five additional scripts follow where water is located in different places. The hypnotherapist has a variety of water features to work with: a birthing pool, a pond, a fountain, a waterfall and a water park. The main theme throughout is relaxation and embedding the idea of water moving down and making time go quicker to help with the birthing process. Additional scripts are included to work on:

- Movement and letting things happen naturally
- Cooling down body temperature
- Energising and feeling refreshed
- Bonding
- Forward pacing.

The script

I wonder where your subconscious mind will go to when I say the word – water. Just think about water. It is one of the basic things we need in life to survive – a real necessity. When you start thinking about it, water has lots of uses and it can help us in so many different ways. Water is a powerful thing – it is a powerful force. I would like you to think about water, because I think it may be of help to you through your pregnancy.

I am going to ask you to imagine certain things related to water – as you keeping drifting deeper into trance – sometimes hearing my words – sometimes not hearing them – it really does not matter. Your subconscious mind is going to hear everything I say.

So, as you relax more and more now – just start to imagine the different places where you might find water. When you come into my therapy room, you know there is always water there – waiting for you – ready to drink whenever you need it. You know that some people find they have a very dry throat when they come out of trance. Water is refreshing – it quenches your thirst – drinking plenty of water is a healthy thing to do. Let's imagine some places where you might find water and use water to relax and help you.

(Guidance note: the hypnotherapist can choose which location/water features they want to use)

DOI: 10.4324/9781003173779-16

Additional script 1: Birthing pool

I know you are looking forward to being in a birthing pool while your baby starts his/her journey into the world. A birthing pool is such a lovely place to be. Just for a few moments now imagine the birthing pool. See it in front of you – look around you – I wonder what you see. Look down into the water – how calm and inviting it is. Just step into the water now. Feel the water – with your hands and your feet. I wonder what the temperature is like – is it right for you? Change the temperature if it needs to be different – warmer or cooler – however you want it to be. Go further down into the water and enjoy the feel of the water against your skin. Walk around the birthing pool – get a feel of it – the size of it. What else might you do in the pool? Sit – lie – float. Explore the birthing pool – imagine what it might be like when the baby is on his/her journey. Who will be there? What will you be doing? See yourself in the pool – enjoying the water – feeling calm – feeling relaxed – feeling excited about your baby coming into the world. Keep feeling and sensing the water all around you – calming and inviting – welcoming your baby into the world.

Additional script 2: Pond

Imagine walking in a park and you see a pond. Look for the different birds that might be in or around the pond – ducks, swans, geese, maybe some herons. All enjoying being in or near the water. See how still the pond water is – very still and very calm. Calm – just like you can be at any time you need. See the birds gliding smoothly through the water – easily – serenely – gracefully – smoothly – just letting things happening naturally. Calm – just like you can be at any time you need. Imagine yourself gliding along the water in the pond – it comes so naturally. Feeling so calm. Gliding forward so gently. So, when your baby starts on his/her journey you can visualise the calm pond. See the ducks and swans gliding along the water in the pond – easily – serenely – gracefully – smoothly – just letting things happening naturally.

Additional script 3: Fountain in the ground

I know a city that has an amazing fountain right in the middle of the city centre. It is not your typical fountain – one that might be built of stone and water runs down different tiers. No, this fountain is completely different. The water comes up out of the ground. When the fountain is turned off – you would not even know it existed.

Just imagine that you are walking in that city centre – along a very busy road. There are lots of people on the pavements either side of the road; lots of traffic on the road travelling in both directions. Suddenly you look to your left and you see a quiet place. There is a bit of greenery and some benches nearby. Then you notice that actually there are lots of places to sit. There are even steps up to seats in what looks like an open-air theatre. Beyond the greenery you see a flat bit of land – it looks like it is made of concrete.

You notice the people who are sitting down are all looking at one spot on the flat concrete. They look very expectant. You wonder what they are waiting for. You look over there too – then suddenly water starts coming out of the concrete. Rising up – lots of little mini fountains coming out of the ground. The water starts getting higher and higher. You cannot believe how high the water is spurting upwards. You are amazed at this different fountain – a fountain that goes upwards.

Suddenly you see a group of children running towards the fountain and then they run through the fountain. Running in and out – in and out. Then some adults do the very same thing – running in and out – in and out. So, would you like to try that? Run into the fountain – feel the coolness of the water – so refreshing – and out again. Run into the fountain again – feel the coolness of the water – so refreshing – and out again.

This time run right into the centre of the fountain and stay there. Feel the refreshing cool water coming upwards – from your feet to the top of your head. Feel the coolness going up through the whole of your body – how refreshing. From your feet up through your legs – your hands and arms – your front and back – your neck – your face. So refreshing you are completely refreshed. The fountain is somewhere to come when you need to cool down and feel refreshed.

Additional script 4: Waterfall

You are walking through the middle of a rainforest. It is humid and hot. You feel hot and sticky and very, very tired. Your body is aching with the heavy tiredness you feel. You feel you cannot go on – you just do not want to walk anymore – you have no energy left at all.

Then you hear the sound of water. That makes you feel maybe you could go on a little bit further just to find the water. Having a drink of water will cool you down. Having a drink to quench your thirst. You walk towards where you think the water might be. The sound of water running gets louder – you walk a bit quicker – you need to reach the water.

Then you see it. A beautiful waterfall. Water falling down so quickly. Thick and fast. The water is falling down and down and down. Walk towards the beautiful waterfall, and feel some of the coolness coming from the falling water. Walk a little further and walk into the water. That feels so great – cooling your feet – walk nearer to the waterfall. Let your hands play with the water. Feeling cooler now as you are nearly in the waterfall.

In you go – immerse yourself completely in the waterfall. Feel the cold water coming down – down onto your head – your face – your neck – your arms – your hands – your front – your back – your thighs – your calves – your feet. Enjoy the cold water coming down – making your body cooler and cooler. As your body becomes cooler you do not feel tired anymore – instead you feel pleasantly relaxed and also energised in a very invigorating way. Keep enjoying the feeling of the cold water coming down and down and down – you feel relaxed – energised – ready to carry on your journey when you are ready to do so. For now though, just keep standing in the waterfall – enjoy the cold water – feeling relaxed and energised.

Additional script 5: Water park

Imagine that you are having a day out at a water park. It is a beautiful summer's day – a perfect day for swimming and playing in water. This water park has so many different things in it for you to explore. Imagine that you are walking up to the entrance. Maybe you can hear water running – people laughing, shouting and screaming – they are all having so much fun. There is a bit of a queue to get into the water park, but there are several places to pay the entrance fee so you will not have to wait long – time can pass so quickly when you want it to do so. Pay your money and in you go. It is time to explore.

I wonder what you might see first. There are so many different things – so many places to swim and play. You may see large pool areas. Water slides. Canons shooting out water. Log flumes. Splash pads. Lazy rivers. Each one of these things can help you in their different ways. Think about the power of water – the power to help – such a force.

There will be times in your pregnancy or when you are birthing when you might get hot and need to cool down. Just imagine being very hot in the water park now – dripping with sweat. Hot and uncomfortable. Walk towards one of the areas where there are huge canons shooting out ice cold water. Stand in front of the canons and feel the rush of the water coming at you – cooling you down. How fantastic. The water keeps coming – you are cooling down – getting to just the right temperature that you need to be. Cooling – cooling – cooling you down. It feels so good. The power and force of the cold water is helping you get to the temperature you need to be – just right – perfectly comfortable.

Maybe you would like to take a rest now – go on a restful, peaceful journey. Go and find the lazy river. As you are walking, notice all the other facilities you might come back to in the future. The splash pads – where water springs up out of the ground – another place where you can cool down. All the different places to take a slow, relaxing swim.

You will find the lazy river in a short while. You will see a number of rafts tied up waiting to be taken by customers. There is no queue at all, so find a raft you would like to use. Someone will give you a hand onto the raft – as it sways gently on the water. That's right, on you go. I wonder if you will choose to sit or lie down on the raft. Do whatever is most comfortable for you. Now that you are settled the person who helped you get on the raft will untie the raft.

Close your eyes and just feel the gentle sway of the water. The raft starts to drift – feel the gentle sway. The raft is moving forward and starting its journey down the lazy river. As the raft moves forward you feel a sense of laziness yourself. A laziness in the positive sense – just relaxed and not a care in the world. There are no pressures at all – you do not have to do anything and you do not have to think about anything at all. Just a time to be lazy and enjoy your surroundings and your journey down the lazy river. Travelling lazily, gently, no rush at all. You have all the time in the world to take your journey down the lazy river. Lazily and gently – all the time in the world. Feel the gentle sway as the raft travels forward on the lazy river.

After you have finished your journey down the lazy river, you might like to experience another type of journey. Why don't you find a water slide? A water slide that you would like to travel down very, very quickly. One that would give you the experience that times passes so quickly. Find the water slide you would like to travel down.

Climb up the steps to the very top. Climbing up towards the beautiful clear blue sky. You feel like you are climbing to the top of the world – it is so high. You feel excited about the journey you are about to take – down the slide. When you reach the top of the steps there are two people waiting in front of you. Feel the anticipation – your excitement is increasing. The person at the front sits down and starts down the slide. Your excitement is increasing even more. The second person now sits down and starts down the slide. It is nearly your turn.

You step forward and look down. It seems a long way down. The slide has lots of twists and turns in it. Are you ready? Take a deep breath and sit down. Ready, steady and go – start your journey down the water slide. Feel the water under your legs as you start to slide down. Twisting and turning. Going faster and faster. Enjoy every moment. Feel water splashing on your face – your arms – body and legs. How exciting is this? You take each twist and turn confidently – nothing frightens you. You deal with every unexpected twist and turn. You can deal with whatever you have to face next. Your body adjusts – it knows what to do. Down and down – twist and turn. Time is going faster and faster. Faster and faster. You are nearly at the bottom now. A few more twists and turns. Prepare yourself to come off the water slide and into the pool. Whoosh – there you go.

After all that excitement you might like to go for a gentle swim now. Just relax. Nice even strokes – swim at a pace that is good for you. Swimming can be so relaxing but it also such very good exercise for you and your baby. And whilst you are taking this gentle swim perhaps you would like to imagine your baby swimming with you – swimming inside of you. Your baby sees, feels and hears what you do. Your baby is swimming gently in the womb. Talk to your baby now.

(Guidance note: if working with a group the hypnotherapist can have a few minutes silence so mum can swim with the baby. In individual sessions, more in-depth work can be undertaken with regard to talking and bonding with baby as mum swims)

Water can be so relaxing. Feel the gentle ripples of the water moving away from you as you continue to swim. The water is keeping you afloat – so supportive – so gentle on your skin. The water is making you feel good – relaxing you. As you relax more with each stroke that you take – imagine the future with your baby. Imagine when you take him/her to a swimming pool for the first time. Carrying your baby into the pool – introducing your baby to the water. Then imagine your baby as a small child – taking swimming lessons – wearing arm bands – using a float. Imagine your child playing on a beach and then running into the sea and swimming. Imagine your child as a teenager – growing up so fast – so confident in the water – playing with friends. Time passes so quickly – enjoy and savour every moment with your baby. Whilst you are swimming it is such a good time to think about the lovely things you are going to do with your baby in the future. Just keep swimming and imagining.

Part IV

Practising self-hypnosis and working on issues

17 The practice nest

Introduction

Most hypnobirthing teachers are forever saying to their clients 'Practise. Practise. Practise' – and that is very good advice. Some mums will take it very seriously and practise rigorously, others might be a bit more laid back and others might find it incredibly difficult to fit in the practice to their busy daily lives. The idea behind creating the practice nest is to give mum a place to go in her imagination where she can practise her breathing techniques or do absolutely nothing – just relax. It can be really helpful to mums who find it difficult to discipline themselves and practise self-hypnosis on a regular basis. The hypnotherapist can suggest setting a goal to visit the practice nest at least once a day.

The practice nest is a place to return to in future sessions. Other scripts in this book can be used as stand-alones but many of them, designed for practising techniques or working on specific issues, work really well when using the practice nest as a starting point.

The script

You know that your imagination can take you anywhere you want to go. You also know that you need to practise your breathing every day in order to prepare for the arrival of your baby. So, it would be good to have a particular place where you could go to practise.

I want you to imagine that you are standing out in the open somewhere and you are surrounded by trees. If you look upwards you can see the clear, blue sky; and maybe some birds flying very high. Look how smoothly those birds are flying. Their wings flapping up and down in perfect rhythm – up and down. The wings look small but in fact they are incredibly strong and so very powerful. The birds can fly to wherever they want to go.

I wonder if you have ever thought about what it might be like to fly like a bird. Just start walking forward – being aware of everything around you – the trees – the birds – any sounds you might hear. You feel relaxed and calm, but also a little excited. Just quicken your pace a little – not much energy is needed. You still feel relaxed and calm.

Now walk a little faster – and a little faster – and even faster. It is almost as though you are preparing to take off. So, go as fast as you need to lift yourself off the ground and fly like a bird. Up you go – just flying naturally – up and up and up – as high as you can go. Enjoy flying around – still going higher and higher – up and up. Enjoy your flight.

DOI: 10.4324/9781003173779-17

As you are flying around look at the trees – all different shapes and sizes. Notice the trunks of the trees – the branches – and the leaves. Keep flying around – in and out of the trees – until you see a nest in one of the trees. Tell me when you see it. Good. Now fly towards the nest and then when you reach it land gently and safely. Just sink into the nest. Sinking down – feeling so soft and comfortable.

This nest is where you can come to practise all the things you have learnt in order to prepare for the birth of your baby. Just keep sinking down into the nest – feel as though you are moving through the floor of the nest. That's right. Keep going down and down – and as you go through the floor of the nest, you will start to see that the nest has different rooms. These are rooms you can visit at any time. Each room will serve a particular purpose for you. I do not know what rooms you are going find because only you know what you need. So just pause for a moment and think about some of things you have thought about, discussed and prepared for in regard to your wellbeing, pregnancy and arrival of your baby:

*   Taking time out for you
*   Going into trance
*   Breathing
*   Visualisations
*   Mantras/affirmations
*   Eating healthily
*   Exercising
*   Bonding with your baby.

(Guidance note: the hypnotherapist may wish to insert their own topics they have worked on with mum at this point. The idea is for mum to find rooms where she can do these particular things/tasks)

Is there anything that you need to do?
Is there anything else that you want to do?
Is there anything else that is important to you?

OK – so now start looking around the nest and find the rooms you need. You can make these rooms just as you want them to be. So, start exploring and tell me what you find.

(Guidance note: it is important not to lead mum as she needs to create her own rooms but some rooms might be:

*   *Kitchen*
*   *Bathroom*
*   *Bedroom*
*   *Nursery*
*   *Playroom*
*   *Quiet room*
*   *Study/reading room*
*   *Gym*
*   *Spa*

The hypnotherapist should work with mum to create each room and decide what she will do in each room, that is, what purpose will a room serve)

18 Dad: you're important too

Introduction

The subject of this chapter is working with a dad. This could be a biological dad or someone who is going to be a stepdad. I do not apologise for this as I think dads sometimes are not given enough attention. There will be all sorts of dads who come to a hypnotherapist because their partner is pregnant. Some will come willingly; others feel it is something they have to do for their partner and a small number will be complete sceptics about hypnosis. The hypnotherapist could have a lot to deal with in relation to dads and I mean that in a good way – it can be challenging but rewarding work.

When running a pregnancy and birthing group, there could be a real mix within a group and this can be a challenge to handle, especially when a sceptic tries to disrupt the group. A dad may be very quiet and uncommunicative because he does not really want to be there; and this could be for any number of reasons. The hypnotherapist needs to use skills to get dad on board and to do this will probably have to do an individual session to find out what is really going on with dad. I always welcome the opportunity to be able to work with a dad in a session which is just for him. Many dads feel they are not important because they believe mum and baby are the only ones who matter. Some dads say they feel redundant. Other dads have specific issues that need attention and therapy.

Below are different sorts of dads who may present with a variety of problems that the hypnotherapist may need to work on; and certainly, this list is by no means exhaustive:

- Young dad: very nervous; knows nothing/little about babies, pregnancy, birth; lacks confidence; unsure of his role and responsibilities.
- Dad who is a dad already: has children from a previous relationship or other relationships; is not really welcoming of the current pregnancy; feels burdened; worried about his financial situation; worried about how his other children will accept the new baby.
- Dad who has lost a baby/child previously: through a miscarriage, stillbirth or childhood death; baby/child taken into care; baby/child put up for adoption; no contact/access denied to child.
- Stepdad is in a relationship with mum but is not the biological father: he may have doubts about his role, capabilities and feelings for the baby.

One of the major pieces of work which needs to be undertaken with dad is regarding his role and responsibilities in relation to the pregnancy and birthing process. Many

DOI: 10.4324/9781003173779-18

scripts in this book can help with that, but in addition other issues could come to light; some of the major areas to work on can be in relation to:

- Anxiety
- Fears/phobias
- Stress.

Using benefits therapy[1] in hypnosis can be very powerful and I think it is very useful when working with dads. Some dads may feel threatened by the imminent changes which are about to occur in their life when a baby arrives. Rather than worrying about the negatives it can be helpful to focus on the benefits of the situation. Some of the scripts written for mum can be adapted for use with dad, but as I have already said I think it is good to be able to offer dad some individual attention. The hypnotherapist can work with dad as s/he would with any client who has a specific issue to address. What follows below is a general script I have written for dads, which focuses on re-laxation, remaining calm, considering his roles and responsibilities but specifically utilising the concept of benefits.

As explained elsewhere in the book, I will get mums and dads (or birthing partners) into trance altogether in a group session. In individual sessions I will also get mum and dad into trance together. This is so that dad can learn self-hypnosis himself and practise getting into trance as well as mum. I also create a safe place for dad and will usually use the finger and thumb technique to anchor. The following script assumes that dad has already learnt some basic techniques and has created a safe place he can go to for relaxation and to practise. It is imperative that the hypnotherapist allows sufficient time to let dad think and to work in depth with responses he gives.

The script

Close your eyes gently. Make yourself comfortable in the chair. Just imagine you are sinking deeply into the chair. Keep your breathing slow and steady. Remember the simple number breathing technique you have learnt. Breathe in – *1, 2, 3* – and hold. Now breathe out slowly – *3, 2, 1* – relax. Good and again. Breathe in – *1, 2, 3* – and hold. Now breathe out slowly – *3, 2, 1* – relax. So, keep breathing slowly as you know how to do and with each breath that you take feel yourself sinking further down into the chair. Down and down.

We have already discussed how today's session is all about you. Focussing on you will benefit you, but it will also benefit (*mum's name*) and the baby. They will feel the benefits that you gain too. Everyone will benefit.

You are relaxing more and more now. Letting everything go. Anything that you brought into the room today – any worry, concern – from home or from work – just let it all go. That's right. Feeling more and more relaxed as your eyelids feel heavier and heavier. You have experienced trance before – you know how good it feels – you know how helpful it can be to let both your body and mind relax. Do that now – relax – and as you go deeper double your sense of relaxation. Good – keeping going deeper and deeper – leaving everything behind – nothing to worry about. Becoming totally relaxed.

Now put your finger and thumb together and go straight to your safe place. Tell me when you are there. What are you seeing? Has anything changed? Do you want to change anything? Do you need to bring anything into your safe place? Remember you can make your safe place just as you want it to be. You can make changes and bring anything or person in at any time.

I would like you to find somewhere to sit in your safe place – somewhere comfortable where you can think, ponder and reflect. So, you are going to be a dad. I think that is wonderful – it can be something to look forward to but I know sometimes it can feel a bit daunting at times. I want you think about the benefits you will gain from being this baby's dad. Do that now – what are you going to gain – what is going to be good about having this baby in your life?

(Guidance note: Dad may very well bring out negative responses initially and the hypnotherapist must work through these before returning to focus on the benefits. Some questions and prompts are given below)

What are you looking forward to?
What will the benefits be of having this baby in your life?
What positive changes will this baby bring to your life?
What are the benefits for other important people/people you care about in your life?
What might you learn from this experience that could benefit you in the future?

Being a dad is a massive role to play in life and this role brings with it responsibilities – some of which might be worrying you. Let's think again about that word 'benefit'. Focus on the word 'benefit'. You have a lot to give of yourself – life experience – knowledge – skills – and your unique personal qualities. You have a lot to give to *(name of mum)*. Think about *(name of mum)* first – and how you can help her through the pregnancy and during the birthing. Think about your life experience – knowledge – skills – and unique personal qualities. Think about/visualise some of your life experiences which you know will benefit you and *(name of mum)*. Think about/visualise your knowledge. Think about/visualise your skills. Think about/visualise your unique personal qualities. Now tell me how you think you can use your life experience – knowledge – skills – and your unique personal qualities to help, support and benefit *(name of mum)*.

(Guidance note: the hypnotherapist should give dad plenty of time to visualise situations and talk about each one he is imagining. The hypnotherapist needs to acknowledge each positive and emphasise the benefits for the future)

Visualise yourself now helping and supporting *(name of mum)*. See all the different ways you can help her during the pregnancy and during the birthing. Look at what you are doing. Hear what you are saying. Tell me about some of the things you are doing and saying.

You see you have so much to offer and so many benefits will be gained. Acknowledge now that you know you have so much to offer and that you can do a good job in helping and supporting *(name of mum)* through her pregnancy and the birthing process.

Now think about the baby. You are going to be his/her dad and from the moment s/he is born s/he will depend on you, look to you for help, advice and this will go on forever. Yes, a big responsibility, but you know you can do it. Think again about your life experience – knowledge – skills – and unique personal qualities. Visualise some of your life experience – knowledge – skills – and unique personal qualities. Now tell me how you think you can use some of your life experience, knowledge, skills and unique personal qualities to look after, help, support and teach the baby.

(Guidance note: the hypnotherapist should encourage dad to talk in depth about what he is visualising. The hypnotherapist needs to acknowledge each positive and emphasise the benefits for the future)

Visualise yourself now with the baby. See all the different things you might be doing with him/her in the first few days of life – over the first few weeks – and then the first few months. Look at what you are doing. Hear what you are saying. Tell me about some of the things you are doing and saying to the baby.

You see you have so much to offer. Acknowledge now that you know you can do a good job in being a supportive partner and a responsible dad. You can help and support *(name of mum)*. You can be part of bringing the baby into the world. Just relax and believe in yourself. Just keep relaxing now – think about all the benefits that you are going to experience during the pregnancy and after the baby arrives. Just relax more and more and focus on the word – benefits.

Note

1 For those interested in reading more about the benefits approach see Chapter 4 in Hunter, R. (2011) *The Art of Hypnotherapy: Mastering Client-Centred Techniques.* 4th edition. Bancyfelin, Carmarthen: Crown House Publishing.

19 Exercising in the gym

Introduction

This script works well with anyone who likes going to the gym. It can be used to focus on promoting physical health and fitness, eating healthily and for practising breathing but it also has four additional scripts to work on other subjects:

- Stretching – imagery for birthing for the birthing journey
- Motivation
- Getting rid of concerns, worries and fears
- Making time go more quickly.

The script

We have previously talked about how important it is to stay healthy and fit during your pregnancy. It is important for you to have a healthy lifestyle as your baby grows inside you. We have discussed exercise and healthy eating, but you may remember we also talked about how your uterus, its muscles and the cervix work through your pregnancy and then how the muscles of the uterus work differently through the birthing journey. So today you are going to visit the gym to do a bit of exercise and to prepare a bit more for your pregnancy and the birthing journey *(or insert a particular topic)*.

Right, so, have a think about what you might need for your work-out in the gym. Imagine what you are going to wear – what you are going to have on your feet. Do you need anything on your head/hair? Now think about what you might need to take with you – a bag – maybe a towel – bottle of water – anything else? Right, are you ready? Yes, you certainly are – ready for some exercise to prepare you for anything that you have to deal with in the future. Acknowledge the mental strength that is embedded deep within your subconscious mind. Feel the motivation and determination deep within you. Feel the physical strength through your body which you are going to work on and increase, so you become fitter and healthier. Feel the inner strength deep within you. Feel the motivation to be fit and healthy. Feel the determination to get even fitter and have a good pregnancy and birthing experience.

Imagine that you have arrived at the gym and that you are standing outside. What does the gym look like? I wonder if it is one of those gyms that has huge glass windows so you can look in and see how people are exercising. Or whether it is more private. This gym is going to be one that suits you best – a place where you feel comfortable. Go into the gym and find the changing room, which will have lockers. If you need to

DOI: 10.4324/9781003173779-19

put anything in a locker, do that now. Take some really deep breaths in preparation for your work-out. Breathe in – *1, 2,* and *3.* Breathe out – *3, 2,* and *1.* As you keep breathing deeply, feel the motivation within you – feel the determination within you – feel the strength throughout your body and also deep within your mind. Feel the motivation to be fit and healthy. Feel the determination to get even fitter and experience a good pregnancy and birthing. Feel *(insert anything else as appropriate).*

Take another deep breath in – *1, 2,* and *3.* As you breathe out, feel the strength in your body and in your mind – *3, 2,* and *1.* Take another deep breath in – *1, 2,* and *3.* As you breathe out feel the motivation to be fit and healthy – *3, 2,* and *1.* Take another deep breath in – *1, 2,* and *3.* As you breathe out, feel the determination to get even fitter and have a good pregnancy and birthing experience – *3, 2,* and *1.* You are good to go.

(Guidance note: the hypnotherapist can then choose which of the following additional scripts may be useful to mum)

Additional script 1: Taking a stretch class

Today you are going to take a gentle stretch class. You will be very good at this as you already know how to control your breathing but, in this class, you can practise your breathing as you are stretching different parts of your body. As you stretch each part of your body remember to breathe in through your nose and then breathe out through your mouth. Just do that one time now – breathe in through your nose and then gently breathe out through your mouth. Good.

OK, so imagine the class has started. There are other women in the room but you are not really aware of them. You are lying on your back – feeling comfortable and prepared. I wonder if you can hear any music. To the count of *3,* you are going to lift one leg at a time as high as you can get it and hold it there for *3* and then gently lower it down for *3.* Then you will do the same thing with the other leg. Ready.

Breathe in – *1, 2,* and *3* and gently lift your right leg slowly and hold it in position. Point your toes to the ceiling for *3 – 1, 2,* and *3.* Now breathe out and slowly lower your right leg to the floor – *3, 2,* and *1.* Now the other leg.

Breathe in – *1, 2,* and *3* and gently lift your left leg slowly and hold it in position. Point your toes to the ceiling for *3 – 1, 2,* and *3.* Now breathe out and slowly lower your left leg to the floor – *3, 2,* and *1.* Now do that again.

Breathe in – *1, 2,* and *3* and gently lift your right leg slowly and hold it in position. Point your toes to the ceiling for *3 – 1, 2,* and *3.* Now breathe out and slowly lower your right leg to the floor – *3, 2,* and *1.* Now the other leg.

Keep doing that in your own time and feel the muscles in your legs strengthen with each lift. Feel all your muscles getting stronger and stronger – stronger and stronger. The more you stretch yourself physically, the stronger you become. It is the same for your mind – the more you stretch your mind, the more positive and determined it will become.

(Guidance note: let mum continue for a short while. Give some positive reinforcement about strengthening)

Now work on your arms – doing a very similar exercise as you did for your legs. You are going to lift one arm at a time so it is up in the air and hold it there. Then gently lower it so it lies behind your head. Then you will do the same thing with the other arm. You will then bring both arms back to their original position. Right, let's go.

Breathe in – *1, 2*, and *3* and gently lift your right arm slowly. Now hold it in a vertical position for *3 – 1, 2*, and *3*. Stretch your fingers and thumb, so they are pointing upwards towards the ceiling. Now breathe out and lower your right arm and take it further back so your fingers and thumb are pointing behind you – *3, 2*, and *1*. Really, really, stretch those arms, fingers and thumb. Now do the same with the left arm.

Breathe in – *1, 2*, and *3* and gently lift your left arm slowly. Hold it in a vertical position for *3 – 1, 2*, and *3*. Stretch your fingers and thumb, so they are pointing upwards towards the ceiling. Now breathe out and lower your left arm and take it further back so your fingers and thumb are pointing behind you – *3, 2*, and *1*. Really, really, stretch those arms, fingers and thumb. Now with both arms stretching behind you, feel those arms, fingers and thumbs stretching as much as they can – stretching away from you.

As you can continue stretching, feel every muscle stretching upwards. Stretching just like the muscles in your uterus will stretch when the baby starts his/her journey. The uterus muscles need to stretch up and up so that your cervix relaxes and opens very naturally to help the baby on his/her journey. Keep imagining the muscles stretching up and up so that your cervix opens very wide and naturally. Stretching those arms up helps the uterus muscles to stretch up. Keep stretching – that's great. Well done. Over the next few weeks and months, you can come back and take a stretch class in your mind and practise stretching your muscles.

Additional script 2: Personal trainer

Sometimes it is good to get some advice and help from someone who is an expert. As you might choose to continue to visit the gym regularly in the future, it might be a good idea to have your own personal trainer. So, make your way to the reception desk in the gym and have a conversation with the receptionist. Explain that you would like to have the help of a personal trainer. The receptionist goes through a door behind the reception area. You need to wait now. Have a think about what you want in a personal trainer – what you need help with – the qualities – the skills – your personal trainer needs to have. You are still waiting at the reception desk. There is no rush – you need to make sure they get the right personal trainer for you. Just be patient – there is no rush. Now in a moment the door is going to open – are you ready? The door will open on the count of *3 – 1, 2*, and *3* – the door opens and your personal trainer is there. Tell me about your personal trainer. What do they look like? Do they have a name? Take some time to chat to them.

(Guidance note: most of the time a human being will appear, but the hypnotherapist should not be surprised if an object appears for some mums. The personal trainer can be used in other scripts to help mum)

Now that you have your very own personal trainer s/he (*or it*) will always be in the gym whenever you need him/her. S/he will be there to help you – advise you – encourage you – motivate you – answer any questions you may have or just listen to you. Your personal trainer will never leave you – they are part of your life – there to help you get fit – stay fit and healthy throughout your pregnancy and for the birthing journey.

(Guidance note: the personal trainer can be incorporated into the following scripts if the hypnotherapist wishes)

Additional script 3: Lifting weights

Something you are worried about or a problem you are facing can feel like a heavy physical weight on your shoulders at times. It can be good to exercise and lift that weight off your shoulders. You have been telling me about *(insert the issue, i.e. worry, concern, problem)* and how it makes you feel. Lifting some weights in the gym might be able to ease the feeling of *(insert what mum has described)*. Imagine that you are in the room at the gym where the weights are located – all sorts of different weights – dumbbells – barbells – all different shapes and sizes. Have a look around – look at the different weights and then choose the ones you would like to use. Pick up the weights in both your hands. They feel heavy – put them down again. You can do this – you can pick up the weights and lift them. If you keep doing this, you will become stronger and the weights will feel lighter. You will feel lighter.

Think about *(insert the issue)*. Pick up the weights again. You are holding them firmly – no hesitation at all. Keep thinking about *(the issue)*. Start to lift the weights – slowly and steadily. They still feel heavy. Lift the weights a little higher – you can do this. You want to get rid of that heavy feeling – you can get rid of that heavy feeling. Lift those weights higher – as high as you can – and then lower them and put them back down. Well done.

Think about *(the issue)* again. This time when you lift the weights you are going to push *(the issue)* away and you are going to feel everything lift from you – you are going to feel lighter – nothing weighing you down. Think about *(the issue)*. Pick up the weights – start to lift them – higher and higher – push *(the issue)* away. Keep going. Lift the weights higher and higher – pushing harder and harder. High as you can and then lower. You are feeling lighter and lighter. But at the same time, you feel stronger and stronger. So now, keep doing that – keep lifting the weights as high as you can and then lowering them. Keep doing that until you feel all the heaviness has gone – there is no heaviness left. Tell me when you are done – when you have pushed *(the issue)* away completely. All the heaviness has gone and you can lift the weights so easily – they feel so very light.

Additional script 4: Pedalling time away

Riding a bike can be good exercise but it can also be good for making time go more quickly – especially when your baby starts his/her journey into the world. In the gym you will find all sorts of different exercise bikes. You could even take a spinning class. For now – find a bike you would like to use and get yourself settled in the saddle. Look at the controls on the bike. You will see a speed dial. You can set your speed – slow – fast – very fast. Why not go for a gentle ride to begin with? Set the dial to slow. Start pedalling – nice and gentle. Just relax – breathe steadily. This is such a good way to get some exercise but also to practise your breathing at the same time. Keep going – pedalling away on the bike – focus on your breathing.

You are in control of this bike. You can do as much exercise as you like – whenever you like. So why not go a little bit faster now – see what you and the bike are capable of.

Turn the speed to 'fast'. You are pedalling faster – you are going to need to concentrate on your breathing – keep pedalling. Keep breathing – control it.

I wonder what is the fastest you can go on the bike. Turn the speed dial to 'very fast'. Pedal even faster now – you are getting faster and faster – you have so much energy – keep going – keep going. Fantastic. Well done. Now turn the speed dial down to 'slow'. Remember you are in control of this bike – you can go at any speed you like. I want you to experiment with the bike now – going slow – faster and very fast, because the bike will be able to help you during birthing. You can make time go more quickly by imagining you are on the bike – you could even drift off on a bike ride somewhere in that great imagination of yours. The bike could take you on all sorts of journeys through the birthing process, but when you want things to move on more quickly you can focus on your pedalling and set the speed dial to fast or very fast and make time go more quickly. So, do that now – practise making time go faster and slower, because when your baby arrives you will want to slow time down and savour every moment. Remember you are in control of the bike – you can make it go faster or slower. Get pedalling now.

20 The bathroom

Introduction

I am aware that many of my pregnant clients love to spend time in their bathrooms. I am often told it is a place they can find some peace and quiet, get away from other people in the home and have some time for themselves. So, it seemed a good idea to write a script located in a bathroom for my pregnant mums. Originally, I wrote a script located in a bathroom with the simple objective of visualising falling water to facilitate down breathing. As with most of the scripts I write, they change and develop over time – usually because of the wonderful imaginations of my clients who inspire me and my own imagination in all sorts of ways. So that is how the bathroom script has evolved over time; it is a place where mum can:

- Relax
- Practise breathing – especially down breathing
- Get rid of things.

The beginning of the script can be used purely for relaxation purposes. I have then used subheadings to divide the script into sections (each having a different objective), so the hypnotherapist can use one or more sections as appropriate.

It must be noted that for some clients the bathroom is not a place they feel comfortable in. I have worked with survivors of abuse who have had very bad memories of incidents which have occurred in bathrooms or have developed phobias about water because of what has been done to them. Also, some male therapists may not feel comfortable using this script with female clients.

The script

I want you to imagine that you are going to have a new bathroom. It is the bathroom you have always wanted. So, on the count of 3 you are going to walk into your beautiful new bathroom – *1, 2,* and *3.* Find the light switch and turn it on so you can see everything very clearly. You are ready to explore your bathroom where you will find many things to help you. So, just start looking around your bathroom.

How many windows are there?

What do you see on the walls? *(e.g. paint; tiles)*

What colours do you see?

Look up and what do you see on the ceiling *(e.g. paint; tiles; type of light(s))*

DOI: 10.4324/9781003173779-20

On one wall there is a cabinet. Open the door and see what you find inside it. There could be all sorts of things that you like but which also could be helpful to you:

- Bubble bath/shower gel
- Moisturisers and oils
- Things you might need when you go to hospital: soap, facecloth/sponge, toothbrush, toothpaste, deodorant.

Can you see anything else?

Tap and washbasin (for deepening and down breathing)

Just imagine walking up to the washbasin. Turn one of the taps on a little bit and see the water start to run. Look at the water running from the tap down into the washbasin and then down into the plughole. Running down – down – down and down. Now turn the tap a little more. The water is going faster now. Watch the water running from the tap down into the washbasin and then down into the plughole. Running down – down – down and down. Turn the tap full on now. The water is going really fast now – gushing into the washbasin and then down into the plughole. Gushing down – down – down and down.

(Guidance note: repeat using the other tap)

The shower (for relaxation and visualising down movement for down breathing)

Find the shower in your beautiful bathroom. I wonder if you have to step into it or whether you walk straight in. Whatever you need to do, go into the shower now. Turn on the shower and feel the lovely warm, relaxing water fall onto your head – run down over your ears – face – throat – and neck. The water is soothing you and relaxing you as it showers you, refreshes you and cleanses you. The water goes down – down – down and down.

You feel the lovely, warm, relaxing water running down one of your arms – from your shoulder to your elbow – down to your wrist – over your hand and fingers and thumb. So warm and relaxing. Down – down – down and down. Then you feel the lovely, warm, relaxing water running down the other arm – from your shoulder to your elbow – down to your wrist – over your hand and fingers and thumb. So warm and relaxing. Down – down – down and down.

Now feel the lovely, warm, relaxing water running down the front of your body. Over your chest and stomach down towards your legs. Down – down – down and down. Now feel the lovely, warm, relaxing water running down the back of your body. Over your shoulder blades, your back and lower back down towards your legs. Down – down – down and down.

The lovely, warm, relaxing water now reaches the top of your legs – running down the front of your legs. Down – down – down and down. At the same time – running down the back of your legs. Down – down – down and down. The lovely, warm, relaxing water continues down and reaches both your ankles. Down – down – down and down. Finally, the lovely, warm, relaxing water reaches your feet and reaches your toes.

Look down now at your feet and watch the water splashing around them and then running away from them. Watch the water as it makes its journey down the plughole. Down – down – down and down. The water is going down – down – down and down.

Turn off the shower. Look down at your feet. Watch all the water go away down the plughole. Down – down – down and down – continuing its journey – down – down – down and down. Keep watching the water down – down – down and down – until all the water has gone. You feel warm, relaxed and refreshed.

The toilet (for getting rid of things, e.g. thought, feeling, fear, worry)

Just imagine now that you are standing in front of the toilet. Whilst you are standing there, I want you to concentrate on your thoughts and feelings. You know that your thoughts and feelings affect your behaviour; and whatever you do influences your thoughts and feelings.

> *(Guidance note: if the hypnotherapist knows that mum has a particular worry or fear this can be substituted for thought/feeling which I have used in the rest of this section)*

If you have any thought or feeling at the moment which is causing you discomfort, I want you to focus on that *(thought/feeling)*. Really *(think about it/feel it)*. When you are ready to get rid of that *(thought/feeling)* – throw it into the toilet. Do that now. Then flush the toilet and watch that *(thought/feeling)* going down the toilet. Watch the water flushing down from all around the toilet bowl – fast and strong – flushing the *(thought/feeling)* away. Keep watching the water flushing down – flushing away – flushing down – flushing away – flushing down until it's gone completely from the toilet bowl. Imagine now that *(thought/feeling)* travelling down the pipes from the bathroom – being flushed down to the drains – being flushed away – deep down into the drains. Travelling far, far, far away – never to trouble you again.

Now that you have got rid of that *(thought/feeling)*, feel that positivity deep within you. You know you can achieve anything you really want to do. You can throughout your pregnancy/during birthing *(insert suggestions as appropriate)*:

- Think positive thoughts
- Remain calm and relaxed
- Be happy
- Be confident
- Be proud of yourself
- Feel excitement
- Feel energised
- Feel joy
- Feel your own strength deep within you
- Enjoy the experience.

The towel rail (for comfort and protection)

Somewhere in the bathroom you will see a towel rail, which is made of strong steel but it has no towels on it at the moment. Stand where you can see it clearly. Just count how many rails it has from the top down to the bottom – and notice how far apart they are.

Now look at the two sides of the rail – right and left. See how long and smooth the side rails are – going from the top of the towel rail down to the floor. Just stand there and feel the gentle warmth coming from the rails. So comforting – gentle warmth circulating around the bathroom – circulating around you.

Now make some beautiful, big, fluffy towels appear on the towel rail. You might want some small ones too but make sure you definitely have some extra big ones. What colour are the towels? Stretch your arms out and touch the towels. Feel how soft they are. Take one of the extra big towels off the rail and wrap it around you. As you wrap the towel around your body, get the feeling of comfort but also you feel safe and protected. Feel comfort – safe and protected. Now take another towel off the rail and wrap it around you. Feel even more comfort – safe and protected.

Any time you feel vulnerable, unsafe or in need of some comfort just imagine the towel rail – make the towels appear – and use the towels to wrap yourself up so you feel comfort – safe and protected.

The shower ball (for stretching during birthing)

Look around the bathroom and see if you can find one of those shower puffs that you can use to wash yourself in the shower. Maybe one is hanging up in the shower or maybe there are some in a cabinet. When you have found one, hold it in your hand. Look at the net materials it is made of – then look at the little rope which can be used to hang it somewhere. Now with one of your hands hold the puff by the rope and let the puff drop down. Look deep into the puff – see the different shapes within the netting. So many shapes and little holes. Now with your other hand pull the bottom of the puff and stretch it down but not too tight. Now imagine that the puff has turned into your uterus. Imagine that your baby has started his/her birthing journey. Imagine you are looking at the muscles of your uterus. Stretch the little rope in your hand upwards – see the muscles stretch upwards – very tight. That is what your muscles do in birthing – stretch upwards as your baby moves down. Stretch those muscles up and tight – open the cervix. Stretch up and tight – good. Stretch up and tight.

21 The healing place

Introduction

The healing place is where mum can come to relax, restore her energy and heal in any way she needs to do – either physically or emotionally – by using the healing hand technique. The introduction to the script involves walking to the healing place and can be used as a deepener. The healing hand is then introduced but can be omitted in later sessions once the tool has been embedded. The healing place can be used with other scripts to deal with specific problems, such as, high blood pressure (Chapter 23, 'Tunnel of calmness'); sleeping difficulties (Chapter 24, 'Sleeping blankets'). In this chapter, I have also included an additional script specifically for morning sickness.

The script

Just close your eyes and make yourself comfortable. Begin to relax as you know how to do so well now. You know how important it is to look after your body that is carrying and supporting your precious baby, but it is equally important to look after your mind. So just relax now – going deeper and deeper – letting go as you breathe deeper and deeper.

You find yourself walking in a deep valley. You are feeling very calm and you start to become aware of your surroundings. On either side of you and far into the distance you see very tall, steep, strong-looking mountains. Look at the different shapes of the rocks on the mountains. You may also see some greenery but you are mainly aware of and sense the strength of the mountains. You feel power and strength coming down from them. You suddenly realise that you feel extraordinarily safe and protected here. It is as though the mountains are protecting you and your baby. You feel different somehow – more at peace than you have ever been. Enjoy this new feeling which surrounds you – the feeling of safety, protection and peace.

Enjoy walking in this deep valley that is surrounded by the very tall, steep, strong mountains. You sense that you are being drawn to a very special place – so just keep walking forward. Taking deep breaths in and out as you go – breathing in the fresh, clean air – breathing out anything that is not good for you or your baby. Keep walking until you see a little pathway that goes down a very slight slope. When you get there just tread carefully down the slope and you will see that the pathway opens into an area where you see a large pool of water and an entrance to a cave. There is water falling down from the top of the cave into the pool of very deep water. You suddenly realise again how different you feel – that new sense of safety, protection and peace.

DOI: 10.4324/9781003173779-21

You become aware of a bright shining light coming down from the top of the cave. The light is so bright it stuns you at first but then you feel as though it is energising you. You have reached the healing place – the place where lots of things can be restored and healed – but also it is simply a place where you can gain energy and light for the wellbeing of both your body and mind. Energy and light can also be gained for the wellbeing of your baby's body and mind.

Now find a comfortable place to sit by the pool of water. I just want you to think about how important it is to take care of yourself – both physically and emotionally. Everyone at some point in their life gets tired and worn down – sometimes to the point where they become physically ill. Even when a person is not feeling ill it is important to still make sure good care is taken of both the body and mind. The body and mind should never be neglected.

You are pregnant – you are not ill. Having a baby is one of the most natural things in the world. You know how important it is to keep healthy and well during your pregnancy. The healing place where you are now sitting is somewhere you can come simply to relax and energise yourself if you need to do so. Being here will help you to maintain your wellbeing and your baby's wellbeing.

There may be times during your pregnancy when you feel tired and as though you have no energy. There may be times in the future when you feel pain – physical pain like having a headache or emotional pain when someone or something upsets you. Any pain can be relieved with the help of a healing hand.

Just let your *(dominant hand)* hover over the water in the pool. Turn your palm downwards towards the water and stretch out your fingers and thumb. Just wait. Start to be aware that your fingers and thumb are beginning to feel different. Just wait. It is as though something is rising up from the water and making your fingers and thumb feel different – a kind of numbness which is actually very pleasant. Just keep enjoying that sensation rising up from the water.

Now you start to feel your hand being drawn down towards the water. Slowly your arm lowers – you are not forcing it to lower – it is just happening naturally. You are just allowing things to happen very naturally. Your arm is dropping down very slowly – lower and lower towards the water. As it drops lower and lower, your fingers and thumb go into the water and gradually your whole hand is immersed in the water.

Your hand feels completely numb now – so very different to your other hand. Just focus on your hand which is in the water and feel the healing powers from the water being absorbed into your hand. Healing powers that can heal physical or emotional pain any time you need it to do so. Feel the healing powers transferring into your hand now. The hand was feeling numb – but now the hand feels different again – it is full of healing powers. Remember from this day on your *(dominant hand)* is your healing hand.

Whenever you feel physical or emotional pain in the future just place your *(dominant hand)* on wherever the pain is located and you will feel the healing powers working – getting rid of the pain completely. Your healing hand has the power to heal both your body and mind. You need to know as well that you do not have to be in any physical pain to use your healing hand. It can be used simply for soothing and comfort.

So, when you are ready, gently bring the hand out of the healing water. As it comes out of the healing water it goes back to feeling like it normally does – just like your other hand. Now place your healing hand on your baby and feel the soothing and comfort – your baby is experiencing the soothing and comfort too. You both enjoy the sensation of soothing and comfort. Use your healing hand any time you like – it is always there – it will never leave you.

And as you are enjoying this experience just return your attention to the bright light streaming down from the top of the cave. The light is now moving towards you, so you are basking in its brightness. The light is full of energy and goodness. It can energise you – restore you – empower you. Feel the light being at its most powerful – full of energy and goodness. Remember any time you need it to do so, it can energise you – restore you – empower you. All you have to do is say 'light' to yourself and you will feel that light bringing you the energy and goodness you need for you and your baby.

Additional script 1: Swooshing and cleansing for nausea/morning sickness

You have already seen the mountains that surround the pool and cave in the healing place. Nearby there is a spring running with water, which has very special cleansing powers. I know that you have been experiencing nausea/morning sickness. Your healing hand could help with that but I think you would also benefit from visiting the spring. So, come away from the cave and pool in the healing place – come back up the slight slope and you will know which direction to take. Keep walking and again enjoy that feeling of safety, protection and peace from the mountains that surround you. Keep walking until you find the spring. Tell me when you get there.

Look at the water that is running in the spring. It is absolutely crystal clear – it is pure. The water has very special powers to cleanse thoroughly and get rid of bad things. What is very unusual about this water is that it has no taste at all. Somewhere near the spring you will see a cup – go and find the cup now – tell me when you have found it. Can you describe it to me?

Dip the cup into the spring and fill it to the top. Hold the cup tightly in your hands. I know this will be a bit unpleasant but I want you to remember the last time you felt nauseous/sick or you were actually sick. Just imagine how you felt then. Stay with that feeling and now take a gulp of water from the cup. Feel the water in your mouth – remember it does not taste of anything – it is very pure. Swoosh the water around your mouth – do that several times – concentrate on the swooshing. Now swallow the water.

The special powers in the water are going to cleanse your body. The water is going to find whatever is causing you to feel nauseous/sick and swoosh it or them away. Imagine the water travelling around your body – swooshing and cleansing – swooshing and cleansing. Swooshing away the nausea/sickness and cleansing your body so you feel good again. Focus on the crystal clear, pure water – just looking at it in the cup helps you to feel better. Maybe you want to take another gulp of the water from the cup. The swooshing and cleansing continue. You are starting to feel better – the nausea/sickness is going. Keep drinking from the cup – swooshing and cleansing until the nausea/sickness has gone completely and you feel well – really well – ready to get on with the rest of your day.

If the nausea/sickness returns at any time in the future, just say the word 'cup'. Imagine the spring, fill the cup with water from the spring, drink from it and start swooshing and cleansing.

22 Body scanner

Introduction

I have found over the years using the body scanner script to be a really effective way of building confidence and giving reassurance, especially when a client has a tendency to worry a great deal and or has a pessimistic attitude. Where a client does have problems, which may be physical or emotional, the script helps the client to verbalise what they see as the problem and what might be a solution. I need to be clear this script is *not* to be considered a medical diagnosis. The objective is to enable the client to identify what they believe to be the problem. What usually happens is a lot of the session is spent focussing on emotional issues, which may be manifesting themselves physically. Work is undertaken on how the client sees things, that is, their perception, and then to make positive changes for the future. Clients usually feedback that they find the body scanner very insightful and powerful; and the shift in emotions is very immediate.

This script should be used with an individual (i.e. mum, dad or birthing partner) but should not be used with anyone who is claustrophobic or who has been locked away at some point in their lives (e.g. abuse victims; people who have been trafficked). It is useful, but not imperative, to have used the healing place script beforehand so the healing hand technique is already in place for use if required.

I have also included an additional script to facilitate seeing and talking with the baby. The body scanner can be used simply to get to the womb.

The script

Somewhere in the room you will see a door to what looks like a very big wardrobe. The wardrobe is much taller than you are and the door is wide enough for you to go through very easily. Tell me what else you notice about the wardrobe. Now this is a very special wardrobe because when you are inside it, you can see all sorts of things and it can help you to see things more clearly too.

When you are ready, I want you to walk over to the door. Tell me when you are there. On the count of *3*, I want you to open the door and go into the wardrobe. *1, 2,* and *3* – in you go and shut the door behind you.

You will see that you are in a space – a very safe space. There is plenty of room above your head – and all around you – so you can move about freely. You will see that there are four sides surrounding you and a ceiling above you.

On one of the sides, you will see that there is long mirror. Just turn around, stand back and look at yourself in the mirror. Now look above the mirror and you will see

DOI: 10.4324/9781003173779-22

what looks like a camera but in fact it is a scanner. This is a very special scanner because it can see right inside you. Only you can use the scanner – only you can see what the scanner sees. It can scan the whole of your body to check how everything is working. It can scan to look at your physical body but it can also scan to sense your emotional state and check on your wellbeing. The scanner is there to help you with your wellbeing – make you feel good – inside and outside *(insert additional feelings if appropriate)*. If anything needs a bit of attention it will show you.

Step back now so you are standing against the side directly opposite the mirror. Make yourself comfortable. You do not have stand to attention like a soldier. Just re-lax all of your body – maybe give your shoulders, arms and legs a shake. Relax as you know how to do and keep relaxing your mind – going deeper and deeper – experience a wonderful sense of relaxation.

If you look to the right of you – you will see a light switch. If you look the left of you – you will see a cord hanging down from the ceiling. Just turn the light switch off now. The space around you goes darker but you can still see the mirror clearly. Now take a deep breath in and then gently breathe out. You are ready now for your body scan. On the count of *3* I want you to pull the cord on your left-hand side. *1, 2,* and *3* – pull the cord. The scanner is ready to work. Now look into the mirror – you do not see you as you normally see you. You only see the inside of your body – your skeleton – bones – marrow – vertebrae – muscles – organs – veins with blood flowing gently through them.

In a moment you are going to take control and conduct the body scan yourself. Don't start yet. Just think about how you are going to start at the top of your head and slowly work your way down – looking at every single part of you and checking if anything needs attention. You will see and check your skeleton – bones – marrow – vertebrae – muscles – organs – veins and blood. All the way down to your toes.

You will know if something needs attention because you will see it in the mirror. Otherwise just enjoy the scan – knowing that things are working well – working well together and in harmony. Of course, you can stop and chat with your baby as you go along. Just take your time – there is no need to rush.

(Guidance note: if the hypnotherapist is using the script primarily for mum to talk to her baby it is at this point the additional script 1, 'Talking with baby', should be used)

Now on the count of *3* start your scan – *1, 2,* and *3*. Tell me when you have done the scan – you have reached your feet. Take your time. There is no need to rush.

So how was the scan?

What did you see?

Does anything need attention on the inside?

What needs to be done?

(Guidance note: if the hypnotherapist prefers s/he can talk to the client as they do the scan, i.e. stopping if anything needs attention. Some prompts might be as follows:

Where are you now?

What do you see?

How are feeling?

Does anything need attention?

Is there anything you would like to do; change; feel; say?
Talk to your baby now/for a while
What would you like to say to your baby?
Would you like to ask your baby anything? Remember baby knows best.
How does your baby respond?
Tell me about your baby.

The hypnotherapist should then work with mum on anything that needs attention.
Usually, the subconscious will know what needs to be done and mum will be able
to express this after the scan, but the hypnotherapist also has the option to use
the script 'The healing hand')

Good work. Now I want you to do another scan on the inside of you but this time I want you to scan your emotions. See how you are feeling. You have already scanned your physical being, now you need to scan your emotional being, because your wellbeing is made up of both your physical health and emotional health. Do that now – start scanning your emotions – *1, 2,* and *3.* Tell me when you have finished.

So how was that scan?
What did you see regarding your emotions?
How was your wellbeing?
Does anything need attention regarding your emotional state?
Does anything need attention regarding your wellbeing?
What needs to be done?

(Guidance note: if needed, the hypnotherapist should then work with mum on her
emotions and wellbeing)

Now turn to your left and pull the cord again and look at the mirror. You can see the usual you – the outside of you. Once again you are going to scan your body – looking at the outside. You are going to start at the top of your head and slowly work your way down – looking at every single part of you and checking if anything needs attention. You will see and check your head – ears – face – eyes – mouth – neck – shoulders – arms – hands – trunk of your body – your back – your legs and feet. All the way down to your toes.

So how was the scan?
What did you see?
Does anything need attention on the outside?
What needs to be done?

(Guidance note: the hypnotherapist should then work with mum on anything that
needs attention)

Additional script 1: Talking with baby

Now on the count of *3* start your scan – *1, 2,* and *3.* Take a good look at the inside of your head. See your brain – your subconscious mind is working well with you. Always remember the power of your subconscious mind. You can achieve anything you really want to do *(insert appropriate affirmations for mum or embed some of the following).*

• Remain calm and relaxed
• Be confident

- Be strong
- Leave fear behind you
- Be positive
- Be a loving and caring mum.

Continue your scan – down and down you look at the inside your:

- Eye sockets
- Mouth
- Under your tongue
- See all your teeth
- Inside your throat
- Down your right arm – to your elbow – to your wrist – and now inside your hand – fingers and thumb
- Down your left arm – to your elbow – to your wrist – and now inside your hand – fingers and thumb
- Moving down inside the top of your body – over your chest
- Look for your organs which are working so well
- Your heart is pumping away just as it should
- Your liver – kidneys – bowel – intestine.

Now look for your baby. Find your ovaries – the uterus, and there s/he is – your baby.

How does your baby look?
What do you see exactly?
What is s/he doing?
How do you think s/he is feeling?
Now talk to your baby.

23 Tunnel of calmness

Introduction

This script was written primarily for mums who experience high blood pressure (hypertension) during pregnancy. The main aim is to relax mum by taking her on a calm journey through a tunnel, which is actually her body. The journey facilitates relaxation, promotes calmness, the reduction in tension and shows mum how well her body is functioning. The script teaches a number of techniques including how mum can speed up or slow down time, which can be used during birthing. She also learns how to get rid of the symptoms associated with her own high blood pressure. The script can be returned to in future sessions. It is also useful as a deepener at the beginning of a session.

Two additional scripts are included. The first one, 'Meeting baby', can be inserted when mum is travelling around her body; it enables mum to visit her baby during the journey and assists further bonding. The second additional script, 'The half white circle gauge', introduces a specific technique using a gauge to reduce high blood pressure, which can be used in the hypnotic state or in the conscious state at any time.

The script

You are standing very still. Look straight in front of you and you see what looks like the entrance to a tunnel. Above the entrance you see a sign which says: 'Tunnel of calmness'.

If you look in front of the entrance you will see a boat – floating on some kind of liquid. It is not water – it is a liquid that is thicker than water. The boat is tied up by a rope – waiting to take you on a smooth journey into the tunnel. So make your way towards the boat and step onto it. Untie the rope and sit down. There are two oars in the boat – oars which will take you in the right direction to have a smooth journey into the tunnel of calmness.

So while you are settling yourself on the boat, I want you to think about a few things. You know that there is very close link between your physical being and your emotional being. Your subconscious mind is part of your physical body but it is also an entity in its own right. Your subconscious mind affects how your physical body is – the state of your physical body – how it functions – how it reacts. I know you believe in the power of your subconscious mind and you know that your subconscious mind can change the way things are. Your subconscious mind can change the way your physical body is and how it is reacting. So this can be very helpful when you are pregnant. An example being – your blood pressure can rise or fall. When it becomes high you need to

DOI: 10.4324/9781003173779-23

become calmer. You need to relax. You need to get rid of any negative thoughts, worries or concerns that are causing your blood pressure to rise. So the tunnel of calmness is going to help you relax – it is going to reduce the tension in your physical body – your blood pressure is going to be reduced.

You are in the boat – ready to enter the tunnel of calmness. Put the oars in position – so they are ready to work. You will control the oars – you can tell them how fast or slow you want them to go. Choose whether you would like to sit or lie down in the boat whilst you take this journey. Make yourself really comfortable. Take some really deep breaths – nice and slowly – and relax – ready for your journey into and through the tunnel of calmness.

Now tell the boat to start its journey – the boat moves slowly and gently towards the entrance of the tunnel and then it floats smoothly into the tunnel. You are feeling calm as you look around you. As the boat enters the tunnel you see various shades of blue all around you. Up above you on the ceiling – on the walls either side you. Beautiful shades of blue.

When you look down to look at what the boat is floating on – you see a liquid – it is not water – it is thicker than water – and then the liquid turns bright red. This is the red river which will help you on your journey to calmness. You are going to take a journey – floating on the red river which circulates all around your body – keeping you well – keeping you alive. Keeping your baby well – keeping your baby alive. You want the red river to flow and circulate smoothly – continuously. So imagine the boat moving through the tunnel of calmness. As you take a journey through the tunnel of calmness, your mind and body will absorb the blueness – the calmness that is all around you.

As the boat travels smoothly forward, you are still aware of the blueness around you. As you travel further forward you become aware of some images in the far distance. I wonder where you are – in a leg – an arm – your stomach – your back.

Remember you can tell the oars in which direction you want to travel and where you want to go exactly. You are in control. Maybe you would like to travel down the inside of one of your legs. Have some fun – see what it feels like to travel down your leg. Why not see how fast you can travel – go as fast as you like – feel the excitement of being in control of speed – how fast you can make something happen. But you can also slow things down. When you have had some fun speeding things along, tell the oars to slow down – that's right. Slow the boat right down. So now go in the other direction – very slowly – travel up the leg. Have some more fun – going up and down that leg for a while – go fast and slow – control the speed. Enjoy the journey – no matter whether you are going fast or slow – you are very calm – and always in control.

(Guidance note: leave a bit of time for mum to experiment being in control of speeding things up and down)

So now imagine the boat is travelling up the inside of one of your arms – travelling smoothly. Enjoy the smoothness and calmness. Travelling up towards your shoulder – across your shoulder. Look at what you can see – bones – muscles – all strong and in good working order.

Travel down now – down through your neck – travelling down and down. Feeling more and more calm. Being aware of what is surrounding you in the tunnel of calmness. Seeing the different shades of blue and seeing through the blueness images in the distance. All parts of your body – working well – working smoothly – just as they should. Below the boat the red river is flowing smoothly and as it continues to flow you feel calmer and calmer.

Now in the distance you see a heart pumping – strongly and regularly. The heart is an essential bit of equipment in the tunnel of calmness. The heart keeps the red river flowing – keeping you and your baby well – keeping you and your baby alive. Travel towards the heart and see the ventricles going into the heart. See clearly the heart pumping – feel the strong beat – regular and reliable. Now tell the boat to travel through the heart – feel the strength – feel the regularity – feel the reliability – pumping – beating – feel the strength – feel the regularity – feel the reliability. Feel calm in the knowledge that your heart is working well – just as it should.

Now float in whichever direction you might like to go. Maybe you would like to look at some of your other organs – check in on them – see how they are working.

(Guidance note: leave a bit of time again for mum to enjoy the journey.
If the hypnotherapist is using this script more than once, s/he might want mum to visit
the baby at this point and use additional script 1)

As you are carrying on your journey through the tunnel of calmness – feeling very calm, I want you to think about the high blood pressure you have been experiencing. The tunnel of calmness is a place where you can come to help with this – reduce the tension in your mind and in your body.

I want you to think about times when you have known that your blood pressure has been high. You have told me that you sometimes feel *(insert symptoms mum may have experienced, e.g. pounding in heart or chest, dizziness, light-headedness)*. Whilst you are feeling safe in your boat, imagine those feelings again now. The boat starts to rock from side to side. The red river becomes rough – making waves through the tunnel. Keep with those feelings – I know it is hard – but stay with them for a little while longer. Feel the boat swaying side to side – going up and down. See the red river getting rougher and rougher – see waves appearing – and then getting higher and higher.

Now say very calmly and assertively: 'Stop rocking – be calm again'. Immediately the boat stops rocking and swaying. The red river is smooth and calm – the waves have disappeared completely. You feel completely calm and you know that your blood pressure has been reduced. All those horrible feelings have disappeared. You are calm and feeling well.

Sometimes your heart might start to beat too quickly. This is only natural when you are shocked or have a surprise; or when you are scared or anxious about something. Your heart can also beat very quickly when your blood pressure is high. So let the boat take you back to your heart – go there now. Imagine that you see the heart beating very fast – just look how fast it is beating. Look at the red river flowing very quickly through the ventricles and into the heart. Look at the heart again and tell it to slow down. Do that now – slow down your heart. Good.

You are ready to continue your journey – a smooth calm journey – knowing that you are in control. You can change anything you want – direct the boat in any direction you want to go. As you travel through the tunnel look at the blueness around you and you will absorb its calmness – all the calmness that surrounds you in the tunnel. Tell the oars to start working again – to take you forward in the tunnel of calmness.

As the oars start to work again and the boat moves smoothly forward – look at the blueness around you – enjoy the calmness – absorb the calmness. Remember your mind can change the way your body is and how it reacts. Let your body continue to relax – all the tension from your body has gone. You can come back to the tunnel of calmness any time you want to get rid of any tension or to slow things down – or simply to become calmer. By taking a journey in the boat on the red river through the tunnel of calmness you will become calmer and calmer and calmer.

Additional script 1: Meeting baby

So perhaps you would like to go and see your baby. Tell the oars to take you through the tunnel of calmness, along the red river to your baby who is safely tucked away in your uterus. You see your baby in the distance – all curled up – look at his/her head – ears – shoulders – body – arms and legs. Your baby is safe, protected by the uterine wall. See the muscles keeping the baby safe in the uterus. Take the boat closer and see the umbilical cord and the placenta. The boat is floating on the red river taking you closer. The red river is flowing smoothly just as it should be – bringing you and your baby closer – bringing calmness to your baby. Get the boat as close as you can and spend some time with your baby. Talk to your baby as both of you absorb more and more calmness from the tunnel.

Additional script 2: The half white circle gauge

I want you to imagine a white circle which has a black ring going around the outside of it. Now I want you to remove the bottom half of the white circle, so you are left looking at the top half of the white circle. Look at the black line you can see around the half white circle that is left behind. A straight black line going along the bottom. Then follow the black line around the rest of the outside of the half white circle.

Now bring you attention to the black line at the bottom of the half white circle. Look to the centre of the black line. A pointer will appear. A pointer that can reach to the edges of the half white circle, but for now it is pointing straight upwards – to the centre of the top of the half white circle.

Now look again at the half white circle. Divide the white half circle into three sections by putting a black line in between each section. Good.

Now some words are going to appear – one word in each section. Look to the section on the left – you see the word 'low'. Now look to the middle section – you see the word 'moderate'. Finally look at the section on the right – you see the word 'high'. Suddenly the high section turns completely black. Now look at the moderate section. Suddenly that section turns grey – a very dark grey to the right of that section then there are different shades of grey as you look at that section from right to left. At the very left of that moderate section you see a very light shade of grey. The section on the left – the low section – remains pure white.

Think about when your blood pressure is high. Think about how it affects you – how you feel *(insert symptoms mum may have experienced, e.g. pounding in heart or chest, dizziness, light-headedness)*. Remember the last time your blood pressure was high. Remember how it affected you – how you felt. Watch the pointer move as you remember – where does it stop – in which section?

Now imagine that you are in your boat with the oars travelling through the tunnel of calmness. Absorb the calmness as you travel smoothly on the red river. Feel the calmness spreading through your mind – spreading through your body. Feel and absorb the calmness.

Look back at the half circle. See the pointer start to move – watch it move and tell me when it stops. Which section is it pointing to now?

Whenever you are in the conscious state and you need to feel calmer in order to reduce your blood pressure, imagine the half white circle. You can even do this with your eyes open – you do not have to have your eyes closed. See where the pointer is pointing to – and then move it towards the low section and immediately you will feel calmer – your blood pressure will reduce.

24 Sleeping blankets

Introduction

Many pregnant women do experience sleeping problems later on in pregnancy as they become bigger in size and the baby may not want to sleep when mum does. Mum may be feeling very tired but just cannot get to sleep easily. She may also have lots of thoughts going around her head. I am sure we have all experienced times in our lives when we cannot get to sleep even when feeling excessively tired, and the more you try the wider awake you become.

The script which is presented below is to help mum get to sleep if she is experiencing such problems. Some women find it more difficult to get to sleep at certain times of the day so consequently I developed two versions of the script – one for daytime and one for night-time. I tend to use both in a first session, but mum may choose to use just one in the future. This is a good script for dad/birthing partner to read to mum, which helps mum but also gets dad/birthing partner involved in a very practical and supportive way. Again, it is another way of getting dad more involved as well as helping to resolve a problem. It can also be used to help mum rest during the birthing.

Furthermore, the script is valuable for after the baby has arrived. No matter how tired mum might get, she could find it difficult to get to sleep when she has the chance to do so, such as, when baby is sleeping. Using the sleeping blankets will enable her to get to sleep quickly and grab some rest when the opportunity arises.

The script

I know you have been having trouble sleeping lately. As the baby grows you expand and you have more weight to carry, so your bones and muscles can feel tired, painful and achy – but remember they are doing a good job of supporting you and your baby. I understand it can be hard to get comfortable *(insert any specific problem(s) mum has talked about in relation to getting to sleep).* You know you can practise going into trance and drift to anywhere you want to go in order to relax, but maybe it would be helpful to imagine something new to help you get off to sleep.

I want you to slow your breathing down – start relaxing as you know how to do very well by now. That's good. Breathing nice and slowly. Imagine that you are sitting on the bank of a river. You are starting to feel very peaceful as you watch the river flowing in front of you. Look at how the river flows so naturally – just getting on with things as though it has not got a care in the world. Flowing naturally and easily – not forcing anything to happen.

DOI: 10.4324/9781003173779-24

As you continue to watch the river flowing, look at the water. Look at the colour of the water and feel even more peaceful. Look at the patterns you can see on the surface of the water as it keeps flowing naturally and easily – you are feeling even more peaceful now. Watch how the river flows – feel the flow of the river – making you feel more and more peaceful. So peaceful that you just want to lie down now on your back. Stretch out on the riverbank – that feels so good – as you sink into the grass on the riverbank. Continuing to feel more and more peaceful.

(Guidance note: the hypnotherapist can now use one or both of versions of the script which follows)

Daytime

So now you are lying so comfortably on your back – you are feeling so very peaceful and relaxed. It is daytime. The sun is shining brightly and you can feel the warmth of the sun on your skin, which is just so relaxing.

Just think about the sun high in the clear blue sky – not a cloud to be seen anywhere. Lots of people think the sun is yellow. A true fact is that the sun is actually white – it is a mixture of all the colours of the rainbow: violet – indigo – blue – green – yellow – orange and red. When it is time for the sun to set it might seem like the yellow sun has turned orange or red. All very beautiful colours. I wonder what colour the sun is to you now. Does it seem yellow or is it some other colour?

Think about the sunshine; feel the sunshine that comes down from the sun. Rays of sunshine which come down directly from the sun – feel the warmth. Imagine the rays now – whatever colour you choose. Look again at the sun high up in the blue sky and look at the rays coming down – moving slowly and gently. Moving down towards you on the riverbank and as they do so, you feel the gentle warmth on your skin again.

The more you concentrate on the rays of sunshine coming down from the sun you start to feel very sleepy. It feels as though the rays of sunshine are melting away any thoughts you have in your mind. Those intrusive thoughts which will not let you rest are just melting away in the warmth of the sunshine. Melting away in the warmth of the sunshine. The rays of sunshine are making you feel really sleepy now – sleepier and sleepier.

The rays of sunshine are coming down towards the riverbank – see the sun's reflection on the water. Moving slowly – the rays of sunshine are almost reaching the water – almost there now. You keep feeling the warmth which is making you feel even sleepier and sleepier. The rays of sunshine are moving along the riverbank and in a moment, they are going to wrap around you like a warm blanket – so comforting.

The rays of sunshine have reached the riverbank now. The warm rays of sunshine are spreading out on the riverbank – to the left and to the right. Feel the rays of sunshine hanging over your body – feel the warmth coming down making you feel sleepier and sleepier. Now feel the rays of sunshine wrapping around you – the rays of sunshine are wrapping you up ready for a very deep sleep. The rays of sunshine are your sleeping blanket – wrapping you up – ready for a very deep sleep. You feel comfortable and ready for sleep wrapped up in your sleeping blanket. So now keep feeling that warmth and comfort as you drift off to sleep – just drifting – drifting off for a very deep sleep.

Night-time

So now you are lying so comfortably on your back – you are feeling so very peaceful and relaxed. It is night-time. The moon is full tonight, looking big and shining brightly in the black sky. You can also see lots of stars sparkling all across the black sky.

Just think about the moon high in the black sky. Lots of people talk about the silvery light from the moon. The moon itself is actually white but sometimes looks yellow. Start to turn off the stars now – do it one by one – making the sky darker as each star is turned off – and the moon becomes even brighter. As you turn off each star you start to feel sleepy – sleepier and sleepier as the sky goes blacker and blacker. Go on – keep turning off all the stars – you are feeling sleepier and sleepier.

Now all the stars have been turned off, think about the moon and the moonshine. Look at the moonshine coming down from the moon high in the sky. Feel the moonshine that comes from the moon – feel its warmth. Imagine the moonshine now – I wonder what colour it is to you. Look again at the moon high up in the black sky and look at the moonshine coming down – moving slowly and gently. Moving down and as it does so, you feel the gentle warmth on your skin again.

The more you concentrate on the moonshine coming down from the moon, you start to feel very sleepy. It feels as though the moonshine is warm and melting away any thoughts you have in your mind. Those intrusive thoughts which will not let you rest are just melting away in the warmth of the moonshine. Melting away in the warmth of the moonshine. The moonshine is making you feel really sleepy now – sleepier and sleepier.

The moonshine is coming down towards the riverbank lighting up the water on the river. The moonshine is moving slowly – moving along the riverbank now. You keep feeling the warmth which is making you feel even sleepier and sleepier. In a moment the moonshine is going to wrap around you like a warm blanket – so comforting.

The moonshine is on the riverbank now. The warm moonshine spreads out on the riverbank – to the left and to the right. Feel the moonshine hanging over your body – feel the warmth coming down making you sleepier and sleepier. Now feel the moonshine wrapping around you – wrapping you up ready for a very deep sleep. The moonshine is your sleeping blanket – wrapping you up – ready for a very deep sleep. You feel safe and ready for sleep wrapped up in your sleeping blanket. So now keep feeling that warmth and comfort as you drift off to sleep – just drifting – drifting off for a very deep sleep.

25 Your very own hotel

Introduction

As I explained at the beginning of the book, I believe it is important for a hypnotherapist to use a variety of methods and techniques when using hypnosis for pregnancy and birthing. Even when a mum comes specifically to learn hypnobirthing, other work/therapy may need to be undertaken. In my day-to-day practice I like to use regression techniques to find the root cause of a problem. There are hypnotherapists who do not favour using regression at all and prefer to use other ways of working. When working with pregnancy and birthing, I like to look to the future with mum and whoever is involved in supporting her, but it can also be a crucial aspect of the work to provide some therapy in relation to the past. I developed the 'hotel' script to facilitate working on the past, the present and the future. The hotel can be a safe place for mum to relax, maybe practise what she has learnt but also a place which she and the hypnotherapist can return to in future sessions to continue the therapeutic process.

The main script introduces mum to her hotel (her subconscious) and shows her what is available. The two additional scripts which follow can be used to take mum to the future (the first floor) or go back to her past (the lower floor). When going back to the past, the hypnotherapist should be prepared for the possibility that mum might go back to a past life. I always advise students and newly qualified hypnotherapists to undertake some specialist training in this area to help them develop their use of regression techniques further.

The script

You know already that your imagination can take you anywhere you want to go and going to different places can distract you when needed. Already you have visited lots of places and learnt useful techniques to help you during your pregnancy. Today I want you to imagine that you are going to take a short leisure break. You are going to find your very own hotel, which will have lots of different facilities for you to use in the future. You can return to your very own hotel any time you like. I have no idea what your hotel will be like – everyone likes different things, so it will be very interesting to find out what your hotel will be like, won't it?

So just keep breathing deeply, relaxing more and more with each breath you take. I am going to count to *3* and when I say *3* your very own hotel will appear in front of you and you will be standing outside of it. *1, 2*, and *3* – see your hotel now. Take a good look at your hotel. Look at the entrance into the reception area. Right above the door

DOI: 10.4324/9781003173779-25

you see a big sign: *(name of mum)*'s Very Own Hotel. Tell me what your hotel looks like from the outside.

Now is the time to go in and explore your hotel. It is going to have so many facilities that you will enjoy and because you are the owner of this hotel you can build extensions or create a new area or facility – anything you want or need – at any time in the future. This is a place where you can come to relax – have fun – be entertained. The hotel has several function rooms so it is also a place where you can think about things, make decisions and work on anything that needs addressing.

So, on the count of *3* – go into the hotel and find the reception area. *1, 2,* and *3* – in you go.

Look where the reception desk is. There is no need for you to check in because you are the owner of this hotel and everything in this hotel belongs to you. So just say 'hello' to whoever is on the reception desk and look around the area. What do you see?

Now you need to know that your hotel has three important floors. You are currently on the ground floor – which is your present life. Underneath this floor is the lower floor, which contains your past. Above this floor on the first floor there is your future. There may be other floors higher up that go far ahead into your future.

Stay in the present for now and have a walk round the ground floor. You will see some signs which will tell you what is located on this ground floor: restaurant – kitchen – bar – coffee shop – lounge – television room – function rooms – gym and swimming pool – spa – beauty salon – creche – toilets – some bedrooms – doors leading to the outside areas. If you look through the windows you will be able to see outside – peaceful gardens – a green for playing croquet or bowls – tennis courts – basketball courts – a cricket pitch – a football pitch. Can you see anything else?

This ground floor offers you so many areas where you can come to relax – practise self-hypnosis – think about things – just drift off. Or you can engage in all sorts of activities to exercise and keep you fit and healthy. This is your hotel where anything is possible.

(Guidance note: the hypnotherapist can then choose how they are going to work with mum in different areas of the ground floor to work on the present using other scripts in the book to:

* *Relax (lounge; bedroom)*
* *Practice breathing/techniques (lounge; bedroom; spa)*
* *Work on education (function room)*
* *Work on diet (restaurant; coffee shop)*
* *Exercise (gym/swimming pool)*
* *Forward pacing (television room).*

The two additional scripts below are provided for when the hypnotherapist chooses to work on the past or the future)

Additional script 1: The lower floor – the past

From the reception area in your very own hotel, follow the signs which will lead to the stairs. You will see two doors. One door has 'downstairs' written on it, the other door says 'upstairs'. On the count of *3* go through the door which says 'downstairs' – *1, 2,* and *3.* Go through the door and you see yourself standing at the top of a staircase.

This staircase has ten steps down and is going to take you into a deeper state of relaxation. With each number I say, you will double your sense of relaxation:

10: Take the first step onto the staircase
 9: Take another step down – feeling relaxed
 8: Feel a wave of calmness going through your body
 7: Going deeper and deeper
 6: Another step down
 5: Halfway down the staircase now
 4: Feeling so relaxed and peaceful
 3: Feeling safe and that wave of calmness goes through your body again
 2: Nearly at the bottom now
 1: You are on the last step. When I say zero step onto the lower floor
 0.

Now you have reached the lower floor you see a corridor stretching out in front of you. You are feeling deeply relaxed and experiencing that wave of calmness again – going through your whole body. This corridor will take you back in time so you can look at the past. You are ready to work on *(insert issue to be worked on)*. We are going to ask your subconscious mind to go back in time as you walk along the corridor and find the causal factor of *(the issue)*. Take some very deep breaths and in a moment, you are going to start walking along the corridor. Take those deep breaths and look at the corridor in front of you – look at the ceiling – look at the floor. Like in all hotels, this corridor has lots of doors – both on the right and on the left. You see so many doors stretching far along the corridor.

   This is the corridor of past times. On the count of *3* start walking along the corridor – *1*, *2*, and *3*. Keep breathing slowly and steadily and as you walk along the corridor you start to go back in time – back through this life – very slowly just start going back in time – the last few days – weeks – months – years. That's right. As you walk along the corridor you are going back in time and looking at each door that you pass. Your subconscious mind is going to work with you. You will be drawn to a door that you know you must enter. Just keep walking and tell me when you are drawn to stand outside a particular door.

   Good. Now on the count of *3* open the door and go through it – *1*, *2*, and *3*. Open the door and go in. Become aware of your surroundings. Take your time – just become aware of what you are seeing or sensing.

(Guidance note: the hypnotherapist will now work with mum to talk through the experience, which could be from this life or a past life. The objective is to release the feelings associated with the experience(s). It may be necessary to relive an experience more than once until the emotion/pain is no longer felt. A scaling system of 1 to 10 can be used. Repeating the experience until the feeling is down to zero. Some questions follow which the hypnotherapist may want to use to start the process)

If experiencing an event from the current life:
   What do you see?
   Where are you?
   Is anyone else there?
   How old are you?

What are you wearing?
What happens next?
What is said?
How does that make you feel?
On a scale of 1 to 10 how strong is the feeling?

If experiencing a past life:

Do you know who you are?
Do you have a name?
Are you: male/female; adult/child?
Do you know how old you are?
Do you know where you are?
What are you wearing?
Are you alone or is anyone else there?
Is it day or night?
Can you smell anything?
What happens now?
Go to the next significant event
Go to your death
What happened?
On a scale of 1 to 10 how strong is the feeling?

(Guidance note: usually, when experiencing a past life, events from the life will be faced and then the death will have to be experienced. It is usual to grade the pain – physical or emotional – on a scale of 1 to 10. The client keeps experiencing the death until it is no longer painful [zero] and then the hypnotherapist needs to work with the client to pass over to peace)

Now that you no longer feel the pain of death it is time to move to a peaceful place. Imagine that now. Where are you?

Additional script 2: The first floor – the future

(Guidance note: the hypnotherapist can plan to work on a particular issue/topic and use the rooms on this floor for working on this and then for planning and preparing for the future. Alternatively, mum can be taken to this floor and she can decide what she wants to work on in relation to the future. Mum needs to understand that this floor is for working on the future)

From the reception area in your very own hotel, follow the signs which will lead to the stairs. You will see two doors. One door has 'upstairs' written on it; the other door says 'downstairs'. On the count of 3 go through the door which says 'upstairs' – 1, 2, and 3. Go through the door and you see yourself standing at the bottom of a staircase. This staircase has ten steps going up to the first floor and then it continues up to all the other floors in the hotel. The upper floors in the hotel have lots of rooms and facilities just like the rest of the hotel, but they are different in that they have the facility to help you imagine the future and plan for the future. It might be good for you to take the staircase up to the first floor and start thinking about the future. You have been talking about *(insert issue/topic to be worked on)*. Spending some time upstairs will give you some space and time to think about that more.

Look upwards at the staircase. See what the staircase is made of – look at the ten steps. As you are looking upwards you feel a sense of lightness within you – a sense of positive anticipation. As you climb the staircase that lightness will increase. Anything that has been bothering you or nagging at you will just lift away. You will feel so light. I am going to count you up the staircase and with each number that I say you will feel lighter and lighter. I am going to start counting now.

1: Take the first step. You suddenly feel lighter
2: Take another step – feeling even lighter now
3: It is so good to feel light and airy
4: Just let go of anything that has been bothering you or worrying you
5: Let go of any cares or worries
6: Feeling really light now as you are more than halfway up the staircase
7: Still getting lighter and lighter
8: Ready to imagine the future
9: Ready to plan for the future
10: Ready to face the future. Feeling so very light now.

Now you have reached the landing of the first floor. You see a number of corridors going from the landing. Which corridor would you like to take? Start walking along that corridor and you will see lots of doors on either side of the corridor. Tell me what else you see *(e.g. drinks/snacks machine; recess area with refreshments; other staircases)*. Is anyone else on the corridor?

(Guidance note: the hypnotherapist then proceeds to work with mum on a planned issue/topic or by taking mum's lead. If the former, this can be done by using their own techniques or by using one of the other scripts in the book)

Part V
Preparing for birthing

26 Be prepared

Introduction

Some people are very well organised and will have no need of this script at all because they plan way in advance. Other people may have a tendency to leave things to the last minute or they lead very busy lives so they have not factored in time to think about getting practical things ready for the baby. This script can be used in any session to think about the practicalities of getting a nursery ready, packing a bag for hospital – really giving thought to what might be needed.

I want to urge a word of caution if a hypnotherapist is going to work with a young girl or a group of girls, who may not have much financially or could be living in poverty. Many hypnotherapists will be running pregnancy and birthing groups for women who are financially secure and will not have to worry that they cannot afford to buy things they want for their baby. It is important to be mindful when working with a group that the members may have very different values, for example, some may be very materialistic and think nothing of spending vast amounts of money; whereas others may want to (or have to) make things for the baby themselves. The hypnotherapist could have to deal with some challenging comments and conversations. This again is another reason why I think it is important to screen and assess before bringing people together as a group.

Hypnotherapists like myself may choose to offer group sessions free of charge for people who are struggling to survive and have very little because of being on benefits or in the care system; providing for a baby could be a real problem and therefore any form of support may seem totally out of reach. The script needs to be used sensitively and some preparation work undertaken to ascertain whether there will actually be a nursery or whether the baby will be sharing a room with mum, dad and/or siblings.

The main script is presented below, followed by three additional scripts. The first two focus on preparing the nursery and packing a bag for hospital. The third additional script is aimed at mums who are not well off financially and to embed the belief that they have a lot to give their baby emotionally and that they can be resourceful to meet physical needs. It works well with single mums or very young girls in individual or group sessions and can be beneficial to use in conjunction with the metaphorical script 'Sadie' (Chapter 49).

DOI: 10.4324/9781003173779-26

The script

I do not know if you were ever a girl guide, but you might know anyway the girl guides have a motto, 'Be prepared', which means that a girl guide is ready to cope with anything that comes her way. We have talked about how important it is to practise your breathing to help you remain calm and relaxed and this is preparing you for birthing, but today I would like you to think about being prepared and what else it might mean to you.

So just relax and let your thoughts flow naturally – no need to force them – just let your thoughts come when the time is right. If you can, visualise the motto: 'Be prepared'. That's right – see how the two words are written. In a moment I want you to look at each individual letter – follow the shape of each single letter – go around each letter one at a time. As you look at each letter you will go deeper into trance – deeper and deeper and feel more and more relaxed. Start now going round each letter: b – e – p – r – e – p – a – r – e – d.

Now you are feeling deeply relaxed – more relaxed than you have ever experienced before. You are preparing to welcome your baby into the world, so think about what preparations you need to make, because you want to be fully prepared for when your baby arrives. S/he will come into the world when s/he is ready, because baby knows best – you need to be prepared – s/he might start their journey when you are not expecting it – a pleasant surprise.

You might want to think about things you need for yourself – for your baby – for dad/birthing partner – for your home. You might want to think about things you need to do – like packing your bag ready for hospital. Just let your mind bring forward your thoughts about being prepared.

> *(Guidance note: the hypnotherapist can ask the generic open questions which follow below and/or use the following mini scripts regarding the nursery and packing a bag)*

So what thoughts are coming into your mind?
What do you need to prepare?
What do you need to do?

Additional script 1: The nursery

It is so exciting planning a nursery for your baby – thinking about what you would like to put in it. It does not matter how much or how little is in there – it just needs to be a place where your baby will feel safe, comfortable and loved. Somewhere you can care for and communicate with your baby.

Start seeing the nursery. The room which will be the nursery for your baby.

> *(Guidance note: the questions below are there to facilitate mum into imagining the nursery. The hypnotherapist should encourage mum to describe in detail what she is seeing and ensure she is happy with the way things are)*

Should anything be changed/be different?
Is this how you want it to be?

Look around the walls. I wonder what they are like – are they painted or is there wallpaper or maybe a mural?

What colours do you see on the walls?
Are there any pictures, posters or photos hanging on the walls?
Is there a window? Do you see curtains or a blind or maybe shutters?
What furniture do you see in the nursery? *(e.g. cot; wardrobe; drawers)*
Where will the baby sleep in the future – the first few weeks, months or years?
Is there somewhere for you and baby to sit together?
Is there anything else that needs to be in the nursery? *(e.g. nappies; nappy bin; wipes; creams)*
Is the nursery prepared for your baby?
Do you see any toys or books?
Do you see any clothes?
Do you see anything else?

Just go forward in time now, see you and your baby in the nursery.
See yourself talking to him/her.
See yourself dressing him/her in the morning.
See yourself changing his/her nappy.
See yourself getting him/her ready for bed.
See yourself reading him/her a story.
So now the nursery is ready – the nursery is prepared – you are prepared.

Additional script 2: Packing a bag

(Guidance note: this script has been written for mum but can be adapted for dad who needs to pack his own bag)

You need to pack a bag – ready for when you go to the hospital to birth your baby. You are at home thinking about which bag you will pack and what needs to go in that bag. So, choose that bag now – go and find it. Take the bag and place it on your bed. Now start thinking about what needs to go in that bag. Think about what you need first – you are very important.

Start packing for you and tell me what you are putting in the bag as you go along.

(Guidance note: the hypnotherapist should let mum pack her bag, but the checklist below can be used for prompts if necessary)

- Nightdress/pyjamas
- Dressing gown
- Slippers/socks
- Towel
- Hairbrush
- Toiletries; nipple cream; stretch mark lotion
- Tissues
- Maternity pads
- Things for distraction: book; magazines; music; crossword puzzles; sudoku; games; knitting/crochet
- CDs/tracks for hypnosis

- Clothes for going home
- Copy of birthing plan.

Remember some things will have to go in at the last minute or into your handbag:

- Mobile phone and charger
- Headphones
- Laptop; iPad
- Bottle of water
- Food/snacks.

Now think about your baby. What will s/he need in hospital and for coming home?

- Nappies
- Vests
- Babygros/sleepsuits
- Clothes for going home.

Now think about dad/birthing partner *(if there is going to be one)*. Does anything s/he might use need to go into your bag or might they need a separate bag?

- Mobile phone and charger
- Headphones
- Laptop; iPad
- Camera
- Toiletries
- Bottles of water
- Food/snacks
- Book/kindle
- Scripts
- Prompt cards.

That's good – you have prepared well for your journey to hospital.

Congratulations, you have started your preparations today to welcome your baby into the world and then to bring him/her home. You know that there are a lot of practical things to prepare and you are well on the way to doing that – you know what you want to do. You are also preparing mentally and emotionally. Your subconscious mind will continue to bring thoughts forward to prepare you physically and emotionally for your baby's entry into the world. You know it is good to be prepared. You know you can and will be prepared for your baby. Over the next few weeks and months, you will regularly say to yourself the girl guide's motto 'Be prepared'.

Additional script 3: Material things do not matter

(Guidance note: this additional script can be used in conjunction with the meta-phorical script, 'Sadie' [Chapter 49])

I know you might be worried about not having things ready for your baby and how you are going to manage to buy things the baby needs. I want you to breathe out all those worries. Breathe out hard. Breathe in gently and then breathe out hard – breathe out every one of those things you have been worrying about. You have so much love to give to your baby and that is all that matters.

Just relax now and think of some of the positive things you have in your life now and think of the benefits you are going to have in the future. Think about what you will gain from having this little person come into your life – unconditional love – fun – laughter – hope – and so much more.

It is true we are living in a very materialistic society – so many adverts trying to sell, sell, sell. A lot of things are not really necessities – they are accessories. A baby's needs can be simple. I want you to think about the fact that babies have been coming into the world for thousands of years – and so many of them have arrived into a stark society. Think about the cave men and women – they lived in caves – how they lived – having to go and hunt for food. A baby can survive with basic simple things and lots of love.

You are resourceful. Imagine yourself now planning for the future. Think about what you really need to get for the baby. You do not need designer shops or to spend massive amounts of money. Think about where you can get some bargains – charity shops – buy and sell on Facebook – E-Bay. See yourself finding bargains and being really pleased with yourself. Maybe someone you know has had a baby and does not need their baby clothes anymore and suggests you could make good use of them. I wonder if you could make some things yourself – maybe you could learn to knit or sew. Can you paint or decorate? I am sure you have skills that can be put to good use. You can be creative in so many different ways and make things yourself for your baby – that is so much more personal and special. Things you make or create yourself will be full of love for your baby.

Remember you have so much to give your baby. Do not let other people lead you into a pathway of competitiveness and believing that material things are important. Remember you have so much to give your baby – you can and you will provide for your baby.

27 Birthing plan

Introduction

I have found that parents-to-be have had mixed expectations and experiences in relation to birthing plans. A lot has depended on when they have started to come for
hypnosis. If they attend early on in the pregnancy, they may not have thought about a
birthing plan at all. If they start a bit later on, they may have heard about a birthing
plan but not given any real thought to it. Later in the pregnancy some may have done
some work on a plan in conjunction with another person, such as, the midwife. It all
seems very inconsistent what a mum might be offered in terms of developing a birthing
plan by the medical/nursing professionals. Whatever the situation, it is important for
the hypnotherapist to give the subject of having a birthing plan some attention. I have
often been met with blank looks when suggesting we have a think about this. I can get
a completely different reaction from a mum who has birthed before and maybe not
had a very good experience – she knows exactly what she wants to happen and usually
welcomes the opportunity to talk about it. However, it should not be necessary to have
had a bad experience before thinking about how you would like things to be. It can be
helpful to think in terms of 'do's and 'don't's and develop a list of both which can then
be inserted into the birthing plan.

I want to return to the subject of a mum's past and how undertaking a proper
assessment is so important. A mum may have had a previous bad experience giving
birth, but any aspect of mum's past could affect how she is going to be during the
birthing and what she wants to happen. For example, it is helpful for nursing staff to
know (with mum's consent) if the baby is the product of a rape. Any victim of sexual
assault or sexual abuse may be very wary of any form of touch. Many women find
medical examinations very invasive and intrusive; it is going to be even more so for
a victim of sexual abuse. When setting up a new group for survivors of abuse, my
colleague and I always spend a lot of time discussing ground rules and discussion
of touch takes up a large part of the conversation. For example, we ask if someone
becomes upset during the group meeting what do they want us to do or not do. Many
survivors will say they do not want us to come near them or to touch them, as a natural reaction from many people would be to try to physically comfort someone who
was upset by putting an arm around them. It can be particularly helpful to use this
script in conjunction with 'It is your body' (Chapter 38), when mum does have a fear
of being touched.

Working on a birthing plan can be done in the conscious state or in the trance state.
Where a mum has no idea where to start, I think it is better to do most of the work in

DOI: 10.4324/9781003173779-27

the trance state after an initial chat about how the session will be undertaken; explanation needs to be given about:

- Objective: to think about the birthing whilst in trance
- The needs and wants of mum
- How the hypnotherapist will work, i.e. asking some questions/giving prompts
- The hypnotherapist will be taking notes, which can be written up as a birthing plan after the session.

What follows is a script which will get mum into trance and introduce the idea of a birthing plan; this is followed by a series of questions which the hypnotherapist can use to prompt mum. The same questions are presented in Appendix 27.1, which can be used if the work is going to be done with mum and dad/birthing partner (or surrogate and intended parents) in the conscious state.

The hypnotherapist can choose when to use this script and will incorporate it into the timetable/agenda of the package they are offering a group or an individual/couple. I have placed it in this part of the book to preface the following four chapters which include scripts which are to be used to plan and prepare for the birthing; it is a logical progression in helping the planning process and using forward pacing.

The script

You have heard me say before that it is good to let things happen naturally – there is no need to force things – just relax and let things happen naturally. Life will always bring you new situations to face and deal with. Sometimes it is exciting not to know what is around the corner; at other times it is better to be prepared and have a proper plan in place. That is what I want you to think about today – a birthing plan. I just want you to keep going deeper and deeper into trance so that your subconscious mind relaxes more and more. Your subconscious mind is going to work with you and your baby to help you think about the birthing – how your baby is going to start his/her journey into the world.

It is so important for you to be relaxed and for your baby to be relaxed when the birthing journey starts. You know you already work well together – you are in perfect harmony. So now you are going to think about what will help you to remain in a calm and comfortable state during the birthing journey. If you are calm and comfortable – then your baby will be calm and comfortable too.

In a moment I am going to ask you think about what you want and what you need during the whole birthing process from the start – when the surges begin. To the finish – when the baby arrives into the world. And immediately afterwards. There are lots of things to think about and plan for. Who you want to be there in the birthing room with you or who should not be there. What will be helpful to you – what might not be helpful to you. I want you to think about words and phrases – actions and behaviours. So now just keep relaxing – you and your baby are relaxing together – thinking about birthing together – in perfect harmony. Just let your mind drift – imagine your baby has just started his/her journey into the world. Imagine where you are – what is happening. Your baby is further on in his/her journey now. Just think about how you would like things to be. What is important to you? What should happen? What must not happen? Keep thinking about the different stages of the journey.

As you are thinking about the journey think about anything in particular that you would like to happen or not happen whilst you are birthing.

(Guidance note: some mums at this stage have no problem at all saying what they want to happen and what should be in a birthing plan. What follows below is a list of questions and prompts for the hypnotherapist to use while encouraging mum to visualise what is going to happen. Some questions will not be needed depending on mum's responses)

- So where are you going to give birth? *(e.g. home or hospital)*
- How do you want to travel to hospital?
- Where will you park?
- Who do you want to be with you in the room? *(e.g. dad/birthing partner; children; other relatives; friends)*
- Is there anyone who should *not* be in the room?
- What do you need in the room? *(e.g. food; drink; lighting; candle; smells; music; quiet/silence)*
- What else might be useful? *(e.g. book; CD/track; scripts; prompt cards)*
- Is there anything that should *not* be done? *(e.g. by dad/birthing partner; medical/ nursing staff)*
- Are there any words or phrases that annoy you or irritate you?
- When might you want to be silent/others to be silent?
- Positions for birthing *(e.g. preferences/things that might be tried)*
- Use of touch during the birthing/journey: yes or no (if yes, by whom, when and how)
- How do feel about/what are your wishes regarding:
  - membrane sweep
  - induction
  - vaginal examinations
  - use of forceps
  - caesarean section
  - when the cord should be cut *(e.g. immediately; how many minutes after birth; when it stops pulsating; after the placenta has been expelled)*
  - expulsion of placenta *(e.g. to happen naturally or be managed by injection)*
  - having stitches
  - skin to skin contact *(e.g. immediately after the birth/for how long)*
- Breastfeeding or bottle
- To give baby Vitamin K: yes or no (if yes, how to administer: by injection or orally)
- Anyone who needs to be contacted after the baby has been born.

Well done. You have given a lot of thought to your birthing plan today. Just relax some more now – you deserve some pure rest. As the subconscious mind relaxes it often works even better. So, as you relax more and more, your subconscious mind might think of more things – more 'do's and 'don't's for your birthing planning. For now though, just relax – take some time before coming back to the conscious state. Just relax – until you hear me say your name.

Appendix 27.1: Questionnaire for developing a birthing plan

STRICTLY CONFIDENTIAL

Questionnaire: Birthing Plan

Name of Mum:
Date of Birth:
Address:
Telephone/mobile:
E-mail address:

- So where are you going to give birth? *(e.g. home or hospital)*
- How do you want to travel to hospital?
- Where will you park?
- Who do you want to be with you in the room? *(e.g. dad/birthing partner; children; other relatives; friends)*
- Is there anyone who should *not* be in the room?
- What do you need in the room? *(e.g. food; drink; lighting; candle; smells; music; quiet/silence)*
- What else might be useful? *(e.g. book; CD/track; scripts; prompt cards)*
- Is there anything that should *not* be done? *(e.g. by dad/birthing partner; medical/ nursing staff)*
- Are there any words or phrases that annoy you or irritate you?
- When might you want to be silent/others to be silent?
- Positions for birthing *(e.g. preferences/things that might be tried)*
- Use of touch during the journey: yes or no (if yes, by whom, when and how)
- How do feel about/what are your wishes regarding:
  - membrane sweep
  - induction
  - vaginal examinations
  - use of forceps
  - caesarean section
  - when the cord should be cut *(e.g. immediately; how many minutes after birth; when it stops pulsating; after the placenta has been expelled)*
  - expulsion of placenta *(e.g. to happen naturally or be managed by injection)*
  - having stitches
  - skin to skin contact *(e.g. immediately after the birth/for how long)*
- Breastfeeding or bottle
- To give baby Vitamin K: yes or no (if yes, how to administer: by injection or orally)
- Anyone who needs to be contacted after the baby has been born.

Print name:
Signature:
Date:
Time:

28 A trip to the cinema

Introduction

There are so many different ways to forward pace with a client and work with them to look to the future. This has been made easier over the years because we now have so many screens in our lives nowadays that can be used creatively – television, computer, laptop, mobile phone and iPad. One of my favourites has always been to use a cinema screen and make a film. If I know a client likes films and going to the cinema then this is a good technique to use with them. I have developed a series of scripts using the cinema in order to focus on preparation and rehearsal. First-time parents may not have thought about the little but important things, such as, where is the nearest car park; how much will car parking cost; payment methods available. The scripts can also be useful for parents who have children already and may want or need to have a more prepared experience this time round.

I find that clients often think more about things in between sessions and may change their mind about what they want to happen. I emphasise that they can work and change things themselves. They do not have to wait to see me or for the next session, that is, they can go back to the cinema in between sessions. I like using the cinema individually for mum and dad, because it is another way of making dad feel he has an important role to play in the planning.

Mum (or dad/birthing partner) is the director of the film and s/he is encouraged to edit and produce the film. The director is watching the film as s/he is directing, that is, disassociated, but I find that often the director wants to jump into the film and that is absolutely fine and can be worked with. I do actively encourage dad/birthing partner to become an actor in the film so that s/he gets a real sense of his/her role and responsibilities.

The initial cinema script is short and introduces the client (mum, dad or birthing partner) to their own special, private cinema. It can also be used with a group. Other scripts which follow were written originally for individual rather than group sessions, but the main content of them can be used for groups if required – they are:

- Journey to the hospital
- Birthing room
- Birthing at home.

The main objective is to get mum (or dad/birthing partner) to watch a film. Each film script is quite brief in order not to lead mum. The idea is for her to start thinking about

DOI: 10.4324/9781003173779-28

whatever the subject of the film is. The script then develops so the hypnotherapist can work with mum to plan how she would like the scene to play out in real life. This is forward pacing and good for rehearsal. Mum is encouraged to edit the film as much as she likes until she feels it is right – just as she wants things to be.

The script

It is always good to have something to look forward to and you have got a lot to look forward to in the next few months, haven't you? Sometimes even when you are really excited about something, you can feel a little nervous at the same time. The odd worry or concern might come into your mind. So, it can be good to think ahead and give some thought to how you might deal with something – a person or a situation. I am going to ask you to imagine a place where you can go at any time you want so you can plan and rehearse anything you like.

I want you to imagine that you are going to go to a cinema. You will be the only person there because this is going to be a very special showing of a film. Just let your mind relax and start thinking about going to the cinema. I wonder whether your cinema is a very modern one or whether it is an old-fashioned one. Travel any way you like to the cinema and tell me when you have got there.

Now go in through the door and into the main area. Somewhere you will see the place where people can buy tickets, but you do not need to get a ticket because you are a very important person and the cinema is glad to have you using its facilities. If you need any refreshments help yourself to whatever you want – maybe as a treat – a drink – crisps – nuts – raisins – sweets – popcorn – hotdog – whatever you fancy.

When you have everything you need, make your way down a corridor and find a door that has a sign on it that says 'director'. Behind the door is a very private cinema room which is for the person who directs, produces and edits films. So, on the count of *3* go through the door – *1, 2,* and *3.* Open the door and in you go. Look right in front of you – you will see a huge cinema screen – and there is just one seat in the room. On the back of the seat, you will see your name written – look – *(insert name)* – and underneath it says 'director'. Go and make yourself comfortable in your very own director's chair. Just sink into it and feel very relaxed. If you look around, you will find a remote control which will enable you to switch the cinema screen on and off – and do lots of other things as well. So just get yourself really settled – ready to watch a film.

(Guidance note: it is at this point that the hypnotherapist can use scripts in the following chapters to help specifically with preparation:

- *Journey to the hospital*
- *Birthing room*
- *Birthing at home)*

29 Journey to the hospital

Introduction

This script should be used after 'A trip the cinema' has been used. Two scripts are presented below – one for mum and one for dad/birthing partner. It is important to remember that some mums will be giving birth on their own and therefore some parts of a script relating to dad/birthing partner will need to be omitted.

Script 1: For mum

You see the title of the film come up on the screen, 'Journey to the hospital'. I wonder if you can hear any music playing. The film is starting now. You see a pregnant woman in her home. She is walking about going from room to room. She puts both hands on her back and bends over. You wonder if she is feeling some slight discomfort or whether she is in real pain. She stays bending over for a while and then stands up and starts moving again from room to room.

A person comes in and speaks to the pregnant woman. S/he takes her into a room, helps her to sit down and makes her comfortable. S/he then goes out of the picture and you are just watching the pregnant woman again. The film continues. The person comes back into room and s/he is carrying a bag and a coat. S/he helps the woman get up and puts her coat on. They then leave the home.

Outside there is a car *(substitute 'taxi' or 'bus' if it is known that is going to be the mode of transport)*. The two people get into the car and drive off. The film continues – following the car through the streets – stopping and starting – at pedestrian crossings – at traffic lights – stuck in queuing traffic. The journey continues.

After a while, a hospital can be seen in the distance. The car drives closer and then goes through the entrance gates. The car pulls into a car parking space in front of the entrance doors to the reception area. The two people get out and walk into the hospital. See them go. Then you see the title come up on the screen, 'The End'.

Think about what you have just watched so far in the film. Remember you are the director of the film – the film is your very own production. You can tell the actors what to do in the film. This is your production so you change and edit it any way you want. The film can be any way you want it to be. You are in control. You are the director.

Now press the 'rewind' button on the remote control and go back to the beginning of the film.

(Guidance note: the film will now play for a second time. Some prompts/questions are included in the script for use but the hypnotherapist may prefer to use their own prompts/questions to help mum edit the film)

DOI: 10.4324/9781003173779-29

You see the title of the film come up on the screen, 'Journey to the hospital'. I wonder if you can hear any music playing. The film is starting now. You see a pregnant woman in her home. Take a closer look at that woman – you suddenly realise the woman is you. Keep watching the film. Notice what you do. Notice how you look. You can do things differently if you want to – change anything you want if you think it would make the film better.

You are walking about going from room to room. You put both hands on your back and bend over. Look at your face – see how calm it is. Look at how well you are breathing, putting into practice everything you have learnt and practised during your pregnancy for the birthing. You are ready to bring your baby into the world – you are so well prepared. Stay bent over for as long as you need to do so or maybe you would rather be in a different position. Try things out – direct the film – make things just as you want them to be. Remember this is your film, you can produce the footage any way you want. Just see on the screen that you are looking calm and in control. Is there anything else you need to change at this point? How are you feeling as you are watching yourself on the screen?

Continue to watch the film. Notice what you do. Notice how you look. Remember you can change anything you want. The film continues – you are moving from room to room. *(Dad/birthing partner)* comes in and speaks to you.

(Guidance note: the hypnotherapist should work with the responses mum gives and get her to visualise everything she wants to happen. It is necessary to keep reintroducing the theme of directing, producing and editing the film and embedding the fact that she is in control and things can happen just the way she wants)

What does s/he say?
Is there anything you want him/her to do?
Where do you want to be at this point? *(e.g. room; on a chair/sofa/floor; lying down or sitting up)*
Is there anything you need?
Is there anything you need to do?
Is there anything you need to say?
Does anything need to be different?

Just keeping watching yourself on the big cinema screen. You are doing so well. Look at how calm and in control you are. Breathing steadily and well. The film continues. Watch what happens next.

You decide it is time to ring the hospital to see whether it is time to go there. Who is going to make the phone call? OK – watch what happens and listen to the conversation. Tell me what is being said.

It is now time to get ready for the journey to the hospital.

(Guidance note: the following questions should be used one at a time and the hypnotherapist should encourage mum to talk about what she is seeing on the screen and change anything she wants to be different or does not like)

Have you packed a bag?
Who will go and get the bag?
Where is it?
What is in the bag?
Does anything else need to go in it?

Is there anything else you need for yourself?

What are you wearing?

What have you got on your feet?

Do you want to change what you are wearing?

Do you need a cardigan/coat/jacket?

Does anything need doing in the house before you leave? *(e.g. leave food for the cat; put the bins out; turn the house alarm on)*

How are you looking in the film?

How are you feeling as you are watching the film?

Keep watching the film. Notice what you do. Notice how you look. Remember you can change anything you want.

You are ready to travel to the hospital now. How are you going to travel to the hospital? *(car/taxi/bus)*. Outside the house there is the car *(substitute 'taxi' or 'bus' as appropriate)*. You are getting into the car. Which seat are you sitting in? You stretch the seat belt across your bump. The car starts up and then moves off. I wonder if you have any music playing or if the radio is on.

Tell me which way the car goes. Tell me what you see as the car goes along the different streets.

What do you see? *(e.g. other cars; bikes; people; animals; buildings; shops; houses; road signs; street lights; traffic lights; trees)*

How are you looking?

How are you feeling?

Is there anything you want to change? *(e.g. seat/position in car; route taken for the journey)*

The journey continues. You are almost at the hospital now. You are feeling so calm, relaxed, confident and in control. Ready to help your baby into the world. Ready to welcome your baby into the world. You are feeling calm, relaxed, confident and in control. Nothing to worry about at all. In the distance you see the hospital. What does it look like? What can you see exactly? The car is very near the hospital now – getting near to the entrance gates. Where can the car be parked?

Now the car is parked up and you are ready to get out of the car and go into the hospital. Do that now – take your time – get out of the car and close the door. Take a really deep breath. You are prepared and ready. Take another deep breath – really deep – and then breathe out. Go forward – into the hospital – feeling calm, relaxed, confident and in control. Ready to birth your baby. Then you see the title come up on the screen, 'The End'.

Now press the 'rewind' button on the remote control – back to the beginning of the film again. I want you to watch the film from the beginning when you are at home – to the end when you go into the hospital. I want you to pause the film at any point and change anything if you need to do so. Remember you are the director of this film – you are in control – you can make the film just as you want it to be.

I shall remain silent whilst you watch the film again but if you do pause to edit anything please let me know what is happening. I would be very interested to know what is happening in the film. Then tell me when you have finished and are completely happy with the final version of the film.

From now until you are ready to give birth, you can take a trip to the cinema at any time and watch the film again. Like any remarkable film, it would be good to watch it over and over again. Each time you watch it you will see how you are well prepared, ready, calm, relaxed, confident and in control.

Script 2: For dad/birthing partner

You see the title of the film come up on the screen, 'Journey to the hospital'. I wonder if you can hear any music playing. The film is starting now. You see a pregnant woman in her home. She is walking about going from room to room. She puts both hands on her back and bends over. You wonder if she is feeling some slight discomfort or whether she is in real pain. She stays bending over for a while and then stands up and starts moving again from room to room.

A person comes in and speaks to the pregnant woman. S/he takes her into a room, helps her to sit down and makes her comfortable. S/he then goes out of the picture and you are just watching the pregnant woman again. The film continues. The person comes back into room and s/he is carrying a bag and a coat. S/he helps the woman get up and puts her coat on. They then leave the home.

Outside there is a car *(substitute 'taxi' or 'bus' if it is known that is going to be the mode of transport)*. The two people get into the car and drive off. The film continues – following the car through the streets – stopping and starting – at pedestrian crossings – at traffic lights – stuck in queuing traffic. The journey continues.

After a while, a hospital can be seen in the distance. The car drives closer and then goes through the entrance gates. The car pulls into a car parking space in front of the entrance doors to the reception area. The two people get out and walk into the hospital. See them go. Then you see the title come up on the screen, 'The End'.

Think about what you have just watched so far in the film. Remember you are the director of the film – the film is your very own production. You can tell the actors what to do in the film. This is your production so you can change and edit it any way you want. The film can be any way you want it to be. You are in control. You are the director.

Now press the 'rewind' button on the remote control and go back to the beginning of the film.

(Guidance note: the film will now play for a second time. Some prompts/questions are included in the script for use but the hypnotherapist can use their own prompts/questions to help dad/birthing partner edit the film)

You see the title of the film come up on the screen, 'Journey to the hospital'. I wonder if you can hear any music playing. The film is starting now. You see a pregnant woman in her home. Take a closer look at that woman – you suddenly realise it is *(name of mum)*. Keep watching the film. Notice what happens – what you do – how you respond to *(name of mum)*. Think about what she needs – how you can help her.

You see *(name of mum)* walking about going from room to room. She puts both hands on her back and bends over. Look at her face – she seems to be in some discomfort or pain. What do you do to help her? What do you say? See the change in her. See how calm she becomes. Look at how well she is breathing, putting into practice everything you have both learnt and practised together. You are both ready to bring the baby into the world – you are both very well prepared.

You have a very important role to play in the birth of this baby. Yes, *(name of mum)* will physically give birth but you have a very important role to play too. There are so many ways you can help *(name of mum)*. It is important that you remain calm and relaxed too. You know how to help *(name of mum)* with her breathing and you know it helps to practise your own breathing too – so you remain calm, relaxed and confident in the role you have to play.

What I want you to think about is that you are the director of this film you are watching but you have a part to play in the film as well – you are one of the actors. You can try things out. As this is your film you can direct the actors, including yourself. You can produce the footage any way you want. Just see on the screen that you are looking calm, relaxed and confident.

Continue now to watch the film. As you do so, notice what you do. Notice how you look. Listen to what *(name of mum)* says. Listen to what you say. Remember you can change anything you want. The film continues – *(name of mum)* is still moving from room to room. You come into the room where *(name of mum)* is.

> *(Guidance note: the hypnotherapist should work with the responses dad/birthing partner gives and get him/her to visualise everything s/he wants to happen. If the hypnotherapist is already aware that dad/birthing partner has some worries or is anxious about something in particular, then this should be introduced and worked on at this point in the script. It is necessary to keep reintroducing the theme of directing, producing and editing the film and embedding the fact that s/he has an important role to play)*

How is *(name of mum)* looking?
How are you looking?
How are you feeling?
What does *(name of mum)* say?
How do you respond?
Is there anything you want to do for *(name of mum)*?
Is there anything in particular you want to ask or say to *(name of mum)*?
Is there anything else you should be thinking about?
Is there anything you need to do for yourself?
Does anything need to be different?

Just keeping watching yourself on the big screen. You are playing your role so well. Look at how calm, relaxed and in control you are. Responding to *(name of mum)*'s needs. Both of you are breathing steadily and well. The film continues. Watch what happens next.

It is time to ring the hospital to see whether it is time to go there. You are going to make the phone call. OK – watch what happens and listen to the conversation. Tell me what is being said.

What do you need to tell the person taking your call?
What information might the person need?
What questions does s/he ask you?
What questions do you need to ask?
It is now time to get ready for the journey to the hospital.

> *(Guidance note: the following questions should be used one at a time and the hypnotherapist should encourage dad/birthing partner to talk about what s/he is seeing on the screen and change anything s/he does not like)*

(Name of mum) has already packed a bag. You need to go and get it. Where is it?
Take a look inside the bag. What do you see?
Does anything else need to go in it?
Have you got a bag for yourself?
Have you got your prompt cards/scripts?

You might be at the hospital a while, so is there anything else you need for yourself? *(e.g. water, snacks; book)*
Is there anything you might need? *(e.g. mobile phone; iPad; camera)*
You need to feel comfortable – do you need to change what you are wearing?
Do you think *(name of mum)* might need anything else?
Is there anything you need to do in the house before you leave? (*e.g. leave food for the cat; put the bins out; turn the house alarm on*)
How are you looking in the film?
How are you feeling as you are watching the film?

Keep watching the film. Notice what you do. Notice how you look. Remember you can change anything you want.
You are ready to travel to the hospital now. How do you plan to travel? *(car/taxi/bus)*

(Guidance note: if using a car, establish who is going to drive. Do not make the assumption mum and dad/birthing partner may be the only people travelling)

Outside the house there is the car *(substitute 'taxi' or 'bus' if appropriate)*. You help *(name of mum)* get into the car and then you help her with her seat belt. You get into your seat now. The car is started up and then moves off. I wonder if any music is playing or if the radio is on.
Tell me which way the car goes. Tell me what you see as the car goes along the different streets.
What do you see? *(e.g. other cars; people; animals, buildings, shops; houses; road signs; street lights; traffic lights; trees)*
How are you looking?
How are you feeling?
How is *(name of mum)* looking?
Is there any conversation?
Do you need to ask *(name of mum)* anything to ensure she is as comfortable as she can be?
Just keep watching the film.
Is there anything you want to change? *(e.g. route taken for the journey)*

The journey continues. You are almost at the hospital now. You are feeling so calm, relaxed and confident. Ready to play your role. Ready to help *(name of mum)*. Ready to help the baby into the world. Ready to welcome the baby into the world. You are feeling calm, relaxed and confident. Nothing to worry about at all. In the distance you see the hospital. What does it look like? What can you see exactly? The car is very near the hospital now – getting near to the entrance gates. Where can the car be parked?
Now the car is parked up. You get out of the car and go round it to help *(name of mum)* get out of the car. Take your time. What do you say to *(name of mum)* to help/reassure her? Take a really deep breath – you are feeling confident in your role. You are prepared and ready. Take another deep breath. Go forward with *(name of mum)* – into the hospital – feeling calm, relaxed and confident. Ready to perform your role in the birthing of this baby. Then you see the title come up on the screen, 'The End'.
Now press the 'rewind' button on the remote control – back to the beginning of the film again. I want you to watch the film from the beginning, when you are at home, to the end, when you go into the hospital. I want you to pause the film at any point and change anything if you need to do so. Think about things you might need to say or ask *(name of mum)*. Think about things you need to know. Think about things you need

to do. Remember you are the director of this film – you are in control – you can make the film just as you want it to be.

I shall remain silent whilst you watch the film again but if you do pause to edit anything please let me know what is happening. I would be very interested to know what is happening in the film – how you are fulfilling your role. Then tell me when you have finished and are completely happy with the final version of the film.

From now until *(name of mum)* is ready to give birth, you can take a trip to the cinema at any time and watch the film again. Like any remarkable film, it would be good to watch it over and over again. Each time you watch it you will see how prepared, ready, calm, relaxed and confident you are to play your role.

30 Birthing room

Introduction

The birthing room is a very important place for mum and dad/birthing partner. This is where forward pacing can be used and mum can think about how she would like things to be during the birthing. Two scripts are presented – one for mum and one for dad/birthing partner (if there is one). They should be used in conjunction with the script, 'A trip to the cinema'.

Script 1: Hospital setting – for mum

You see the title of the film come up on the screen, 'Birthing room'. I wonder if you can hear any music playing. The film is starting now. You are in the hospital where you have chosen to give birth to your baby. The film is showing various shots of the hospital from different angles – the outside – the car park for visitors – the main entrance to the hospital – where there are a number of ambulances parked outside. Then some shots of the inside – the reception desk – the shop – the café – the lift area.

You are with *(dad/birthing partner)*. Find your way to the area where you know you need to be – where your baby is going to arrive. Go along the corridors – you know which way to go – you feel certain and positive – you know which direction you are going in. You reach the place where you need to be. You speak with a nurse and she takes you to a room. You go through the door and enter the room. This is where your baby will come into the world. You are feeling slightly impatient because you want to see what happens in the rest of the film, so press the 'fast forward' button on the remote control – press 'stop', then 'play.

You are lying on the bed. *(Dad/birthing partner)* is by the side of the bed. A nurse is in the room as well. Notice how you are looking. I wonder how you are feeling. Fast forward again. The baby is nearly here – the birthing journey is nearly over – the baby is reaching his/her final destination. Notice how you are looking. I wonder how you are feeling. Fast forward again. The baby is here. Look at everyone who is in the room. Notice how everyone looks and what they are doing. Then you see the title come up on the screen, 'The End'.

Think about what you just saw in the film and then think about how you want the birthing to be. Remember you are the director of the film – the film is your very own production. You can direct, produce and edit it any way you want. The film can be any way you want it to be. You are in control.

Now press the 'rewind' button on the remote control and go back to the beginning of the film.

DOI: 10.4324/9781003173779-30

(Guidance note: the film will now play for a second time. Some prompts/questions are included in the script for use but the hypnotherapist can use their own prompts/ questions to help mum edit the film)

You see the title of the film come up on the screen, 'Birthing room'. I wonder if you can hear any music playing. The film is starting now. You are in the hospital where you have chosen to give birth to your baby. The film is showing various shots of the hospital from different angles – the outside – the car park for visitors – the main entrance to the hospital – where there are a number of ambulances parked outside. Then some shots of the inside – the reception desk – the shop – the café – the lift area.

You are with *(dad/birthing partner)*. Find your way to the area where you know you need to be – where your baby is going to arrive. Go along the corridors – you know which way to go – you feel certain and positive – you know which direction you are going in.

What do you see as you are walking along the different corridors?
Is anyone else there?
Do you speak with anyone?
Are you and *(dad/birthing partner)* talking? What are you talking about?
How are you looking?
How are you feeling?
How is *(dad/birthing partner)* looking?
Is there anything you want to change?

Keep walking – feeling calm, relaxed and confident, but also excited about the fact your baby is nearly here. You reach the place where you need to be. You speak with a nurse. What is said?

The nurse takes you and *(dad/birthing partner)* towards a room. You stand in front of the door – somewhere on the door you will see names written on it *(insert as appropriate name of mum and dad/birthing partner)* and baby. The nurse pushes open the door and you enter the room. This is where your baby will come into the world.

Now look around the room and tell me what you see.
What colour are the walls?
Are there any windows?
Where is the bed?
How many chairs can you see?
Is there a sink?
Can you see anything else?
Is there another room? *(e.g. toilet/bathroom)*

Have another good look around the room you are in. Is there anything you want to change in the room? OK, so the room is how you want it to be. Get yourself settled, Unpack your bag. Put things where you need them to be *(e.g. music; book/kindle; magazine; iPad; water/snacks)*. Get everything in the right place and make yourself really comfortable and ready to help your baby on his/her journey.

Now look at yourself on the screen. Look at your face – your body – how you are breathing. Is there anything you want to change? Press the 'fast forward' button on the remote control – when you are ready, press 'stop', then 'play. The film continues.

You are lying on the bed. *(Dad/birthing partner)* is by the side of the bed.
Is anyone else in the room?
Should anyone else be in the room right now? *(e.g. doctor, nurse)*

Do you want anyone else in the room?
What are you doing?
Are you saying anything?

Another surge *(or insert whatever word mum is going to use for a contraction)* starts. Tell me what you see on the screen.

> *(Guidance note: the hypnotherapist will let mum talk through the surge and respond to what she says. If appropriate, the hypnotherapist can suggest mum can edit the film as she is experiencing the surge or generic questions can be asked after the surge has finished. Some of the questions which follow can be altered [e.g. replace dad/birthing partner with nurse/doctor or someone else]. The hypno-therapist may suggest that mum watches several surges as the film is playing)*

Is there anything you want to change in that part of the film?
What have you learnt from watching that part of the film?

Fast forward the film again. The baby is nearly here. You are birthing down.
Who is in the room?
What is *(dad/birthing partner)* doing?
What is *(dad/birthing partner)* saying to you *(or anyone else?)*
Do you need *(dad/birthing partner)* to do anything specifically?
Do you need *(dad/birthing partner)* to say anything specifically?
Do you need anyone else to do anything?
Do you need anyone else to say anything?
How you are looking?
How are you feeling?
Does anything need to be different?

Fast forward again. The baby is nearly here – the birthing journey is nearly over – baby is reaching his/her final destination. The nurse says she can see the top of the baby's head. Tell me what happens next.

> *(Guidance note: the hypnotherapist should work through when the baby is born, emphasising repeatedly how well mum is doing)*

Now baby is here. The nurse places him/her on you. You feel baby's skin next to your skin. What a wonderful feeling that is. Spend some time now with your baby *(and dad/ birthing partner if there is one)* – just the two/three of you. Enjoy this unique and special time. Then you see the title come up on the screen, 'The End'.

Now press the 'rewind' button on the remote control – back to the beginning of the film again. I want you to watch the film from the beginning to the end – from when you go into the hospital, find the birthing room and through the whole birthing process. I want you to pause the film at any point and change anything if you need to do so. Remember you are the director of this film – you are in control – you can make the film just as you want it to be.

I shall remain silent whilst you watch the film again but if you do pause to edit anything please let me know what is happening. I would be very interested to hear what is happening in the film. Then tell me when you have finished and are completely happy with the final version of the film.

From now until you are ready to give birth, you can take a trip to the cinema at any time and watch the film again. Like any remarkable film, it would be good to watch it over and over again. Each time you watch it, you will see how you are prepared, ready, calm, relaxed, confident and in control.

Script 2: Hospital setting – for dad/birthing partner

You have such an important role to play being the birthing partner *(or insert dad, parent, grandparent, friend)*. It is truly an honour that you are going to be part of this incredible experience to see a/your baby come into this world. Although it may be very exciting, I know that some people feel a little bit daunted and worry that they might not be able to do what is expected of them. Sometimes they do not know what is actually expected of them or they have no idea what might happen during the birthing journey. So, I think it might be helpful to imagine what might happen in the birthing room and what role you might have to play.

You see the title of the film come up on the screen, 'Birthing room'. I wonder if you can hear any music playing. The film is starting now. You are in the hospital where you are going to help *(name of mum)* give birth to her/your baby. The film is showing various shots of the hospital from different angles – the outside – the car park for visitors – the main entrance to the hospital – where there are a number of ambulances parked outside. Then some shots of the inside – the reception desk – the shop – the café – the lift area.

You are with *(name of mum)*. Find your way to the area where you know you need to be – where the baby is going to arrive. Go along the corridors – you know which way to go – you feel certain and positive – you know which direction you are going in. You reach the place where you need to be. You speak with a nurse and she takes you to a room. You go through the door and enter the room. This is where the baby will come into the world. You are feeling slightly impatient because you want to see what happens in the rest of the film, so press the 'fast forward' button on the remote control – press 'stop', then 'play.

(Name of mum) is lying on the bed and you are by her side. A nurse is in the room as well. Notice how you are looking. I wonder how you are feeling. Fast forward again. The baby is nearly here – the birthing journey is nearly over – baby is reaching his/her final destination. Notice how you are looking. I wonder how you are feeling. Fast forward again. The baby is here. Look at everyone in the room. Notice how everyone looks and what they are doing. Then you see the title come up on the screen, 'The End'.

Think about what you just saw in the film and then think about how you want to help in the birthing room. Remember you are the director of the film – the film is your very own production. You can edit it any way you want. The film can be any way you want it to be. You are in control.

Now press the 'rewind' button on the remote control and go back to the beginning of the film.

(Guidance note: the film will now play for a second time. Some prompts/questions are included in the script for use but the hypnotherapist can use their own prompts/questions to help dad/birthing partner to produce and edit the film)

You see the title of the film come up on the screen, 'Birthing room'. I wonder if you can hear any music playing. The film is starting now. You are in the hospital where the baby will be born. The film is showing various shots of the hospital from different angles – the outside – the car park for visitors – the main entrance to the hospital – where there are a number of ambulances parked outside. Then some shots of the inside – the reception desk – the shop – the café – the lift area.

You are with *(name of mum)*. Find your way to the area where you know you need to be – where the baby is going to arrive. Go along the corridors – you know which way to go – you feel certain and positive – you know which direction you are going in.

What do you see as you are walking along the different corridors?

Is anyone else there?

Do you speak with anyone?

Are you and *(name of mum)* chatting? What are you talking about?

How are you looking?

How are you feeling?

How is *(name of mum)* looking?

Is there anything you want to change?

Keep walking – feeling calm, relaxed and confident. You know that you are going to be a good, helpful and caring dad/birthing partner. You know that you have prepared well. You know what you need to do – how you can help. You reach the place where you need to be. You and *(name of mum)* speak with a nurse. What is said?

The nurse takes you and *(name of mum)* towards a room. You stand in front of a door – somewhere on the door you will see three names written on it *(name of mum)*, *(name of dad/birthing partner)* and baby. The nurse pushes open the door and you enter the room. This is where your/the baby will come into the world.

Now look around the room and tell me what you see.

What colour are the walls?

Are there any windows?

Where is the bed?

How many chairs can you see?

Is there a sink?

Can you see anything else?

Is there another room? *(e.g. toilet/bathroom)*

Have another good look around this room you are in. Is there anything you want to change in the room? OK, so the room is how you want it to be. Now look at yourself on the screen. How are you looking? How are you feeling? Is there anything you want to change?

Now you are helping *(name of mum)* unpack her bag. Ask her if she needs you to do anything else for her. Then sort out your things *(e.g. scripts; prompt cards; phone; camera; water/snacks)* – put them where they need to be. Get everything in the right place so you feel really prepared for helping *(name of mum)* and the baby on his/her journey. Now press the 'fast forward' button on the remote control – when you are ready press 'stop', then 'play. The film continues.

You are with *(name of mum)*.

Where is *(name of mum)* exactly in the room – is she lying down, standing, walking about?

Is anyone else in the room?

What are you doing?

Are you saying anything?

(Name of mum) starts another surge *(or insert whatever word has been chosen for a contraction)*. Tell me what you see on the screen. Tell me what happens – what you do – what you say.

> *(Guidance note: the hypnotherapist will let dad/birthing partner talk through the surge and respond to what s/he says. If appropriate, the hypnotherapist can suggest dad/birthing partner edits the film as s/he is seeing what happens during the surge or the following generic questions can be asked after the surge has finished. The hypnotherapist may suggest that dad/birthing partner watches several surges as the film is playing)*

Having watched the surge(s) is there anything you would do differently?
Is there anything you would say or not say?
Is there anything you want to change in that part of the film?
What have you learnt from watching that part of the film?
Fast forward the film again. The baby is nearly here. You are watching the final stages of the birthing process.
Who is in the room?
Describe how *(name of mum)* is.
Describe what is happening/what you are seeing.
What is *(name of mum)* saying to you *(or to anyone else)*?
How are you looking?
How are you feeling?
Does anything need to be different?

Fast forward again. The baby is nearly here – the birthing journey is nearly over – baby is reaching his/her final destination. The nurse says she can see the top of the baby's head. Tell me what happens next.

(Guidance note: the hypnotherapist should work through when the baby is born, emphasising repeatedly how well dad/birthing partner is doing, that is, being supportive, helpful and responsive to mum)

Now baby is here. The nurse places him/her on *(name of mum)*.

(Guidance note: if the birthing partner is not dad it will be important for the hypnotherapist to know whether mum wants to be on her own with the baby at this point or whether it is OK for the birthing partner to be involved)

Spend some time now with *(name of mum)* and the baby. Enjoy this unique and special time.
Having watched the baby arrive is there anything you would do differently?
Is there anything you want to change in that part of the film?
What have you learnt from watching the last part of the film?
Then you see the title come up on the screen, 'The End'.
Now press the 'rewind' button on the remote control – back to the beginning of the film again. I want you to watch the film from the beginning to the end – from when you go into the hospital, find the birthing room and through the whole birthing process. I want you to pause the film at any point and change anything if you need to do so. Think again about things you might say or ask. Think about things you need to know. Think about things you need to do. Remember you are the director of this film – you are in control – you can make the film just as you want it to be.
I shall remain silent while you watch the film again but if you do pause to edit anything please let me know what is happening. I would be very interested to hear what is happening in the film. Then tell me when you have finished and are completely happy with the final version of the film.
From now until *(name of mum)* is ready to give birth, you can take a trip to the cinema at any time and watch the film again. Like any remarkable film, it would be good to watch it over and over again. Each time you watch it, you will see how prepared, ready, in control, calm, relaxed and confident you are to play your role.

31 Birthing at home

Introduction

Some mums will choose to give birth at home. The majority will be mums who already have a family and believe it will make life easier being at home and having the family involved in the birthing process. However, some first-time mums will choose to birth at home because they definitely do not want to go into hospital. Script 1 is for mum in order to get her to think about how she might want things to be. I have also written a script for dad for him to feel included, but it can be adapted for anyone who might be supporting mum as a birthing partner. I need to say again, some mums will birth without support. The main objective of both scripts is to do some planning, but also to build confidence and embed the belief of being in control. When using these scripts, the hypnotherapist may find a lot comes out regarding relationships within the family network; and work needs to be undertaken to confront issues and dilemmas, for example, who mum does not want in the house when birthing. These scripts should be used in conjunction with the script 'A trip to the cinema'.

Script 1: For mum

You see the title of the film come up on the screen 'Birthing at home'. I wonder if you can hear any music playing. The film is starting now. You are in your own home where you feel comfortable and safe. It is here that you have chosen to birth your baby into the world.

Look at the big screen and start watching the film. It is *(X)* months until your baby will come into the world. You are walking around your home – thinking about how you would like to give birth. Today you are giving more thought to where you will actually give birth. Of course, because you are in your own home you can wander about from room to room – just as you are doing now. Free to do as you wish. But you are contemplating whether it might be a good idea to prepare one room – a special room in which the baby will actually arrive.

You choose a room and you enter it. You are looking around the room and thinking about some changes you might like to make. You also start thinking about things you will need around you. Things that will help you to feel calm, relaxed and comfortable. You are also giving more thought to how you want the birthing to be. What is important to you.

Does everyone who needs to know – know what you need – know what you want to happen – things you do not want to happen – things you do not want said to you? You are feeling slightly impatient because you want to see what happens in the rest of the film, so press the 'fast forward' button on the remote control – press 'stop', then 'play'.

DOI: 10.4324/9781003173779-31

You are lying on the bed. *(Dad/birthing partner)* is by the side of the bed. Notice how you are looking. I wonder what you are feeling. Fast forward again. The baby is nearly here – the birthing journey is nearly over – baby is reaching his/her final destination. Notice how you are looking. I wonder what you are feeling. Fast forward again. The baby is here. Look at everyone in the room. Notice how everyone looks and what they are doing. Then you see the title come up on the screen, 'The End'.

Think about what you just saw in the film and then once again think about which room you might actually give birth in and how you want the birth to be. Remember you are the director of the film – the film is your very own production. You can produce and edit it any way you want. The film can be any way you want it to be. You are in control.

Now press the 'rewind' button on the remote control and go back to the beginning of the film.

(Guidance note: the film will now play for a second time. Some prompts/questions are included in the script for use but the hypnotherapist can use their own prompts/questions to help mum edit the film)

Look at the big screen and start watching the film. It is *(X)* months until your baby will come into the world. You are walking around your home – thinking about how you would like to birth your baby. Today you are giving more thought to where you will actually give birth. Of course, because you are in your own home you can wander about from room to room – just as you are doing now. But you are contemplating whether it might be a good idea to prepare one room – specifically a room in which the baby will actually arrive.

Which room will you choose?

OK, so go into that room now. You are looking around it.

Are there any changes you might like to make?

Do you want to change the colour of the walls?

Would you like some pictures, photos or posters on the wall – or somewhere else?

Might you move some furniture about?

Or even take some furniture out of the room?

Do you need to bring any furniture into the room?

Would anything else make it more comfortable for you? *(e.g. cushions; pillows; bean bags; candles; incense)*

You also start thinking about things you will need around you. To help you to keep feeling calm, relaxed, confident and in control.

Will you have a book to read? Or maybe some magazines?

Might you want to watch a film or a series of something?

Or is there something else you might like to do? *(e.g. crosswords; sudoku; play games; knit/crochet/sew)*

Do you want to listen to music? What sort of music? How will you listen to it?

Could you do anything else?

OK, so the room is just how you want it to be. You are now giving more thought to how you want the birthing to be and what is important to you. Who is going to be there – in your home – in your birthing room? Does that person/people know:

What you need?

What you want to happen?

What you don't need?

What you don't want to happen?
Which words/phrases you find helpful?
Which words/phrases you find unhelpful?
What you don't want said to you?
Have you explicitly told that person/people what you want and what you don't want?

Have that conversation now. Be really clear. You have the right to ask for what you want and for what you need. It is important that you feel calm, relaxed, confident and in control.

You are feeling slightly impatient because you want to see what happens in the rest of the film, so press the 'fast forward' button on the remote control – press 'stop', then 'play'.

You are in the birthing room. *(Dad/birthing partner)* is with you. Is anyone else with you in the room? Now look at yourself on the screen. Look at your face – your body – how you are breathing.

How are you looking?
How are you feeling?
How is *(dad/birthing partner)* looking?
What are you doing?
Are you saying anything? What are you talking about?
Is there anything you want to change?

Another surge *(or use whatever word has been chosen for a contraction)* starts. Tell me what you see on the screen.

(Guidance note: the hypnotherapist will let mum talk through the surge and respond to what she says. If appropriate, the hypnotherapist can suggest mum can edit the film as she is experiencing the surge or the following generic questions can be asked after the surge has finished. The hypnotherapist may suggest that mum watches several surges as the film is playing)

Is there anything you want to change in that part of the film?
What have you learnt from watching that part of the film?
What is *(dad/birthing partner)* doing?
What is *(dad/birthing partner)* saying to you *(or to anyone else?)*
How you are looking?
How are you feeling?
Does anything need to be different?

Fast forward again. The baby is nearly here – the birthing journey is nearly over – baby is reaching his/her final destination. Notice how you are looking. I wonder what you are feeling.

Tell me what happens next.

(Guidance note: the hypnotherapist should work through when the baby is born, emphasising repeatedly how well mum is doing)

Fast forward again. Now your baby is here. You feel your baby's skin next to your skin. What a wonderful feeling that is. Spend some time now with your baby *(and dad/birthing partner if there is one)* – just the two/three of you. Enjoy this unique and special time together.

After you have spent as long as you need together, does anyone else need to come into the room? If so, bring them in now. Tell me what happens. Then you see the title come up on the screen, 'The End'.

Now press the 'rewind' button on the remote control – back to the beginning of the film again. I want you to watch the film from the beginning to the end – from when you start thinking about birthing at home, preparing the special room and experiencing the whole birthing process. I want you to pause the film at any point and change anything if you need to do so. Remember you are the director of this film – you are in control – you can make the film just as you want it to be.

I shall remain silent while you watch the film again but if you do pause to edit anything please let me know what is happening. Then tell me when you have finished and are completely happy with the final version of the film.

From now until you are ready to give birth, you can take a trip to the cinema at any time and watch the film again. Like any remarkable film, it would be good to watch it over and over again. Each time you watch it you will see how you are prepared, ready, calm, relaxed, confident and in control.

Script 2: For dad/birthing partner

> *(Guidance note: I have written the script as though working with dad, but the terminology can be changed for use with anyone who is going to be the birthing partner)*

You see the title of the film come up on the screen, 'Birthing at home'. I wonder if you can hear any music playing. The film is starting now. You are in your own home where you feel comfortable and safe. A decision has already been taken that your baby will be born at home and it is here that you will help and support *(name of mum)*. You have such an important role to play and there is lot to plan for the birthing at home.

Look at the big screen and start watching the film. It is *(X)* months until your baby will come into the world. You are sitting somewhere in your home thinking about the baby and how s/he will be born here. You are letting your mind drift – thinking about what will actually happen on the day of the birth. Then you start thinking about what you need to do – before the birth – during the birth – and when the baby arrives. How you can help and support *(name of mum)* in the best way you can. You are feeling slightly impatient because you want to see what happens in the rest of the film, so press the 'fast forward' button on the remote control – press 'stop', then 'play'.

The baby has started its journey. *(Name of mum)* is walking around the house. I wonder if anyone else is in the house. I wonder what is going on in the rest of the house. Now *(name of mum)* is lying on a bed. You are right next to her. Notice how you are looking. I wonder what you are feeling. Fast forward again. The baby is nearly here – the birthing journey is nearly over – the baby is reaching his/her final destination. Notice how you are looking. I wonder what you are feeling. Fast forward again. The baby is here. Look at who is in the room. Notice how everyone looks and what they are doing. Then you see the title come up on the screen, 'The End'.

Think about what you just saw in the film and think about what you might have to do to help and support *(name of mum)*. Remember you are the director of the film – the film is your very own production. You can produce and edit it any way you want. The film can be any way you want it to be. You can choose how you want to be – how you want to carry out your role and responsibilities in the birthing process.

Now press the 'rewind' button on the remote control and go back to the beginning of the film.

> *(Guidance note: the film will now play for a second time. Some prompts/questions are included in the script for use but the hypnotherapist can use their own prompts/questions to help dad edit the film)*

It is *(X)* months until your baby will come into the world. You are sitting somewhere in your home thinking about the baby and how s/he will be born here. You are letting your mind drift – thinking about what will actually happen on the day of the birth. Then you start thinking about what you need to do – before the birth – during the birth – and when the baby arrives. How you can help and support *(name of mum)* in the best way you can.

(Name of mum) is walking around the house. She then comes to tell you the baby has started its journey.

Is anyone else in the house?

Is anything else happening in the house?

What do you need to do?

Should you ask anyone to leave?

Do you need to make any arrangements for anyone else? *(e.g. other children)*

Do you need to ring anyone?

What do you need to do for *(name of mum)*?

Has *(name of mum)* got everything she needs?

Do you need to ask *(name of mum)* anything?

Now think about you. Where are the things you need? *(e.g. scripts; prompt cards; camera)*

How are you looking in the film?

How are you feeling as you are watching what is happening?

What are you thinking about as you watch the film?

Do you want to change anything you are saying or doing in the film?

Now press the 'fast forward' button on the remote control – press 'stop', then 'play. The birthing process is now well on the way. You are with *(name of mum)* as she is experiencing more surges *(or use whatever word has been chosen for a contraction)*. Look at yourself on the screen. Look at your face – your body – how you are breathing.

How are you looking?

How are you feeling?

How is *(name of mum)* looking?

What are you doing?

Are you saying anything? What are you talking about?

Is there anything you want to change?

Another surge starts. Tell me what you see happening on the screen.

(Guidance note: the hypnotherapist will let dad talk through the surge and respond to what he says. If appropriate, the hypnotherapist can suggest dad can edit the film. It is important that dad is encouraged to think about what he should say and do. The following generic questions can be asked during and after the surge has finished. The hypnotherapist may suggest that dad watches several surges as the film is playing)

Is there anything you want to change in that part of the film?

What have you learnt about your role from watching that part of the film?

Fast forward again. The baby is nearly here – the birthing journey is nearly over – baby is reaching his/her final destination. Notice how you are looking. I wonder what you are feeling.

Tell me what happens next.

(Guidance note: the hypnotherapist should work through when the baby is born emphasising again the importance of dad's role)

Fast forward again. Now baby is here. How do you look? How do you feel? The baby is placed on *(name of mum)*. Spend some time now with your baby and *(name of mum)* – just the three of you. Enjoy this unique and special time together.

After you have spent as long as you need together, does anyone else need to come into the room? If so, bring them in now. Tell me what happens. Do you need to do anything else? Then you see the title come up on the screen, 'The End'.

Now press the 'rewind' button on the remote control – back to the beginning of the film again. I want you to watch the film from the beginning to the end – from when you start thinking about the role you have to play in helping and supporting *(name of mum)*. I want you to pause the film at any point and change anything if you need to do so. Remember you are the director of this film – you are in control – you can make the film just as you want it to be.

I shall remain silent while you watch the film again but if you do pause to edit anything please let me know what is happening. I would be very interested to hear what is happening in the film. Then tell me when you have finished and are completely happy with the final version of the film.

You have such an important role to play in the birthing of your baby. There is so much to think about. Things to organise – people to organise – arrangements to be made. Things for *(name of mum)* and things for you. Like any remarkable film, it would be good to watch it over and over again. Each time you watch it you will see how you are prepared, ready, calm, relaxed, confident and in control.

Part VI
Bonding with baby

32 Bonding on the beach

Introduction

It is incredibly important for mum to take time out to bond with her baby. Most mums will talk to their bump out loud or silently as they lead their daily lives, but bonding can be increased (and should be encouraged) by making an effort to set specific time aside to do this. The hypnotherapist can work with mum to create different locations to achieve this. What follows is a very simple script where mum can bond whilst lying on a beach. The script can also be used as a deepener.

The script

Close your eyes and start to relax. You know how important it is for both you and your baby to relax and have some quiet time together. You are both very much aware of each other but communicating in different ways is such a good way to get to know each other and prepare for the baby's journey and entry into the world. When you think about it, there are just so many different ways you can communicate with your baby. It's not just about talking – you will sense each other – what you both think – feel – and how you behave. So, I want you to think about this but before you do – just let your mind drift – and let your body start to relax. Let your thoughts drift and relax your mind.

Imagine you are lying on a beach somewhere. There is no-one else around. Just be aware of yourself, your baby, the sea and the sky above you. Focus your attention on how you are feeling as you lie on the sand. The sand is soft like a blanket but at the same time firm and supportive like a bed. It is pliable – so it can move to accommodate your body – making things nice and comfortable. If any part of your body is causing you any discomfort just move it and let the discomfort sink into the grains of the sand. Slowly take a deep breath in and then gently breathe out again. With each out breath just deeply relax that part of your body which is causing you discomfort – feel that part sink down into the soft accommodating sand. Now that body part is feeling comfortable you might like to relax other parts of your body. I wonder where you might start.

(Guidance note: the hypnotherapist should ask mum where she wants to start and then help her to move througvh her body. The following are just some parts which can be used as prompts)

Head: Breathe in and gently breathe out – relax
Neck: Breathe in and gently breathe out – relax

DOI: 10.4324/9781003173779-32

Shoulders: Breathe in and gently breathe out – relax
Arms: Breathe in and gently breathe out – relax
Hands: Breathe in and gently breathe out – relax
Front: Breathe in and gently breathe out – relax
Chest: Breathe in and gently breathe out – relax
Stomach: Breathe in and gently breathe out – relax
Back: Breathe in and gently breathe out – relax
Spine: Breathe in and gently breathe out – relax
Buttocks: Breathe in and gently breathe out – relax
Legs: Breathe in and gently breathe out – relax
Feet: Breathe in and gently breathe out – relax.

Now that your body is so beautifully relaxed just let your mind drift. Not a care in the world. Just you and your baby – relaxing together. Just letting things happen naturally – just as they should do. Like the sea in front of you – the waves moving forwards and backwards – forwards and backwards. So soothing – so very natural. Listen to the sound of the waves as they continue to move – forwards and backwards – so soothing – forwards and backwards.

The sky can be soothing too as it changes naturally through the day and night times. Imagine how the dawn appears every morning – the time when the sun rises to lighten the dark night sky. Look at the colour of the sunrise. During the day the clouds and lots of other things move naturally and freely in the sky. Then in the evening the sun drops – watch the sun dropping lower and lower in the sky. Then see a beautiful sunset – look into the different colours – yellow – red – and orange. The sky gradually becomes darker and darker – and then the nightfall arrives. The sky is very dark almost black. The stars come out naturally and freely – and start sparkling in the sky. All so very natural.

So, you will let things happen naturally too, won't you? Let things happen naturally throughout your pregnancy and when your baby starts his/her journey into the world. Your baby knows what to do – s/he will start his/her journey when s/he is ready. Your baby knows what is best.

Now that you are so relaxed and comfortable – letting everything happen naturally, think about your baby relaxing inside of you.

Imagine what s/he is doing inside of you right now.
Imagine what s/he is thinking inside of you right now.
Imagine what s/he is feeling inside of you right now.
Your baby can hear you.
Your baby can sense you.
Your baby can feel you.

You can communicate with your baby in so many different and creative ways – you will sense what is happening and respond to what is happening through – seeing – hearing – smelling – touching and tasting. Your baby will do the same. You both have natural instincts. You will intuitively know how each other is feeling – you have a natural connection. Sometimes you will talk out loud or at other times you will communicate silently. You can communicate with your baby in the conscious state and when you are in the trance state. By communicating with each other regularly you are building a relationship and making a bond – an inseparable bond.

You and your baby are living and working in harmony. There are so many things you are doing together:

- Breathing in healthy, fresh, clean air
- Your hearts are pumping healthily
- Blood is streaming through your veins
- You move together
- You rest together
- You sleep together.

What else do you think you already do together?
What else would you like to do with your baby through your pregnancy?
What would you like to do with your baby during the birthing?
What are you looking forward to doing with your baby when s/he is born?

As you are so relaxed on the beach now think about what you would like to say to your baby. Take your time and then start talking.

33   Message room

Introduction

The hypnotherapist can be creative in how they use this script, the main objective of which is to focus on bonding with the baby by giving him/her messages. It can be good to do this with people who are shy or find it difficult to express themselves verbally in the conscious state. The script can be used with mum or dad separately; alternatively, it can be used with mum and dad in trance together. I also think it is a really good thing to do with dad on his own, because some dads feel left out and not part of it all, that is, they believe they only have a minor role to play.

The main script is followed by six additional scripts, which offer different ways of communicating with the baby – by talking, writing, drawing, recording and keeping a journal. Additional script 4 focuses on writing affirmations which can be used throughout the pregnancy and added to at any time. In additional script 5 a recording is made of what needs to be said and there is an option for mum or dad to tell someone else how they feel about something and/or what they want to happen. This is a good way of rehearsing a situation where something needs to be said or done but mum or dad is dreading the confrontation. The hypnotherapist may choose to use the message room in several sessions. The scripts can be used in pregnancy and birthing groups, but more in-depth work can be undertaken in individual sessions and hence the reason for including additional questions and prompts.

The script

Communication is such an important part of life. It is especially important to talk about how we feel, so people can understand us but also to tell people what they mean to us. With such busy lives people often forget to commend or compliment someone when they have done something well or have achieved something special. We can express our thoughts and feelings in many different ways but today I want you to imagine creating some messages for your baby *(use 'the baby' if the birthing partner is not dad; 'your baby' is used for the rest of the script)*.

It is always good to talk to your baby when you are in the conscious state, but it can be incredibly helpful to express your feelings when in the trance state too. You can reassure your baby how much s/he is wanted and tell him/her about your hopes and aspirations.

Let your mind keep relaxing – you know how to do this so well now. It comes so easily just to relax and let your mind drift. Keeping breathing steadily and let your mind drift – just drift – keep drifting. Let your mind drift and imagine that your mind

DOI: 10.4324/9781003173779-33

is travelling to find a room you have never visited before. Your mind can travel there any way it wants. Keep drifting – travelling to find a room where you feel you could communicate well and be creative in the way you converse and correspond. Messages can be given verbally or they can be written, drawn or painted on many different things – paper, card, canvas, screens, walls or ceilings. Go and find your message room now. Tell me when you find yourself standing outside the door.

What does the door look like?

What is the door made of?

Is there a handle, knob, latch or some other way to open the door?

On the count of *3* open the door and go into the message room. Ready – *1, 2, and 3* – and in you go to your message room.

Tell me what you see first. Now have a really good look around – you need to find things that are going to help you communicate – create some really meaningful and important messages.

(Guidance note: usually mum/dad will find things immediately as the subconscious will have decided how they are going to create the messages. However, if some prompts are needed, the hypnotherapist can suggest mum/dad looks for some of the things which follow)

You need to find somewhere to sit or stand in order to write, draw, paint or talk *(e.g. desk, table, bar, chair, stool, sofa)*. Now I wonder what else you can find to help you create messages. There may be cupboards and drawers in the room hiding all sorts of useful things for writing, drawing or painting. See what you can find *(e.g. whiteboard, blackboard, easel; pens, pencils, crayons, markers, chalk, paints)*. Remember messages can be said verbally and recording messages is also a good way of saying things when you find it difficult to say something to a particular person. Somewhere in the message room I am sure you will find a mobile phone, iPad or a handy little Dictaphone.

You have found a lot of useful resources already in your message room to create all sorts of different types of messages. I am sure there will be more to be found any time you come back in here. In a moment you might like to create one or maybe two messages, but remember you can keep coming back to your message room to create messages and store them here any time you like.

Before you start creating your messages just relax even more than you are relaxed already. The more you relax the more your subconscious mind will work with you to create meaningful messages. So just go even deeper now – feeling relaxed – even deeper – you know that you can. And as you go even deeper still – start thinking about your baby – things you want to tell him/her. Things that are important. Things that are funny. Things s/he needs to know. Things you hope to do in the future. There could be so many things you want to tell your baby.

(Guidance note: at this point the hypnotherapist can choose which additional script will be used in the session)

Additional script 1: The message jar

You have already discovered that this message room is full of things to help you communicate. Look around you once again and see the drawers, cupboards – all sorts of nooks and crannies – good places to store things. Have a root around and see if you can find a very large, clear glass jar that has a lid on it. It needs to be big. Tell me when you have found it. Good. Now this jar has clear glass because it is important that you can get a good view into it. It will also have a tight lid to keep everything that is placed in it very safe.

This jar is your message jar. It has a very specific purpose – it is for you to store all the messages you would like to give to your baby. You might even like to pass on messages from other people too. In day-to-day life thoughts can come into our heads and we think, 'I must remember to tell so-and-so that …', then we forget. During a pregnancy you will have all sorts of things you might want to tell your baby and maybe already you have been saying them to him/her. The idea of having the message jar is that you can come to this room at any time and take some time – have some quiet time – for you to think of things you want to say to your baby in the present time and also in the future. You can also pass on messages from other important people *(if appropriate add other significant people in mum/dad/baby's life, e.g. children; grandparents; relatives; friends and sometimes professionals/workers)*. All these messages can be put in the message jar and will be stored there forever.

Now might be a good time to write a message and to start using your message jar. So why don't you go and sit somewhere – make yourself comfortable? Just relax – imagine closing your eyes. Just feel your eyelids getting heavier and heavier and as this is happening an important message for your baby will float into your mind. Just let the message float in – no need to force it – no need to rush – as you relax more and more – the message will start to appear. Just relax – wait for the message to appear – it will just float in.

(Guidance note: when working in a group the script has to stay very generic, but when working on a one-to-one basis with mum or dad then the hypnotherapist can ask more specific questions about what is appearing, that is, what the exact message is)

When you know what the message is you need to write it down. Look around you – maybe in the drawers or cupboards and see if you can find some paper and a pen. Now write down your message. Just nod your head when you have done that.

(Guidance note: if working on a one-to-one basis rather than in a group, the hypnotherapist can suggest that mum reads the message to the baby out loud)

Fold the piece of paper into a tiny square. Unscrew the lid of the message jar and put the message into the jar. Now put the lid back on the jar. The message is safe.

Over the next few days, weeks and months, you can come back to this room and write more messages from you or other important people. Sometimes you might also like to come to the room, open the message jar and read some of the messages to your baby.

Additional script 2: Welcome messages for baby

You know how good it feels to be welcomed into places – a warm welcome is so important and makes you feel so good. A warm welcome makes you feel calmer when you have reached a new or strange place, where maybe you feel a bit unsure or uncertain because everything is unfamiliar. Just imagine how your baby is going to feel when s/he arrives into the world. S/he has been cosy and warm inside you for the past nine months – secure and feeling safe deep within your womb. So your baby needs to receive a warm welcome. This is something for you to start thinking about – write some welcome messages for your baby. From you – but I wonder if there is anyone else who might want to send a welcome message.

The message room is a good place to write messages. I wonder where you would like to sit to do this. Get yourself in a comfortable position so you can really relax. Let your subconscious mind go into a deep, deep trance and bring forward what you want to say to your baby when s/he comes into the world. Just go deeper and deeper – think about welcoming your baby. Imagine the baby coming into the world – s/he is here – what do you want to say? Good. Now write that welcome message down and then put it in your message jar.

(Guidance note: the hypnotherapist can encourage mum to write more messages in this session or imagine messages from other important people in future sessions)

Additional script 3: A bit of graffiti

Look around your message room and see the walls that protect the room. One wall will have nothing on it at all and you will see that it is made of brick. Go over to that wall and stand where you can get a good look at it. Glance over the bricks that form that wall. I wonder how many bricks there are. Maybe you would like to start counting the number of bricks you can see – starting at the top of the wall. Start counting the bricks now – from the very top. With each number that you count you start to feel more and more relaxed. Keep counting – becoming more and more relaxed with each number that you say to yourself. Keep counting the bricks. Becoming more and more relaxed.

Now look down at the floor and you see some cans of spray paint – all different colours. You are going to write some positive graffiti on the brick wall. I want you to start thinking about some of the key words or phrases that are going to affirm your beliefs and positive thoughts you have about the pregnancy, the baby and the birthing. Take some time and think about some affirming words or phrases.

(Guidance note: typical words that usually come forward are: trust; hope; peace; believe; protect)

Now go and have a look at the cans of spray paint – see what colours are there. If you need other colours go and have a look in the cupboards to find them. Right – you are ready to spray any words or phrases you want on the brick wall. As you write, say the word or phrase to yourself *(if working one-to-one it can be said out loud)* – feel it become fixed on the bricks – and the power of the word or phrase will become rooted deep within you. Off you go – start writing on the wall. Feel the power of the words you are spraying on the brick wall. The words are fixed forever – feel them rooted deep within you. Keep going until the wall is just as you want it to be.

Step back and glance over the words/phrases you have sprayed on the wall. Now look more closely – read and repeat each word whilst remembering each word is now fixed and rooted – fixed and rooted.

(Guidance note: the hypnotherapist must leave a good amount of time for the words to become embedded before continuing)

Read all the words/phrases again. Feel how strong and powerful those words/phrases are. Just like the brick wall – strong, powerful and sturdy – holding up the ceiling of the room. Feel the strength of each word.

Like all good graffiti artists, you need to put your tag on the wall. Think what you might draw as your tag and then spray it on the wall. So, the wall is finished for now, but you can always come back and spray on more words and phrases. At any time in the future, you can imagine the brick wall and read the words and phrases fixed on it. You can do this when you are living your daily life in the conscious state – all you have to say to yourself is 'Graffiti'.

Additional script 4: Message board for affirmations

You know that using affirmations or saying mantras can be helpful throughout pregnancy and during birthing. Affirmations are what you believe in and what you believe to be true. Saying them to yourself every day or seeing them written up somewhere are really good ways to motivate yourself. Your message room is a good place to think about the affirmations you may have developed already but also to develop some new ones. Because you will want to affirm different beliefs as the pregnancy progresses and your baby is growing and developing.

Somewhere in the message room you will find a noticeboard on one of the walls. I do not know what kind of noticeboard it will be or what it will be made of but what I do know is that it will be large enough to put plenty of post-it stickers on it if you need to do so. Find the noticeboard now. Look what shape it is – what it is made of – what colour it is.

Find somewhere comfortable to sit in your message room – a comfy chair or sofa. Just sit down and relax – make yourself really comfortable. Relax – imagine closing your eyes. Feel your eyelids getting heavier and heavier and as this is happening allow your subconscious mind to bring forward your beliefs – think about how you want to live your life. Think about yourself – your part in the pregnancy – the baby – your part in the birthing process – being a parent – and anything else that is important for you and your baby.

As your subconscious mind is bringing forward those beliefs you will start to think about some affirmations – positive statements – statements which will motivate you and you will use during the next few days, weeks and months. Take some time now – no need to rush those thoughts and beliefs. Focus on your beliefs and create some positive statements. Test them out – say them to yourself *(or out loud if working one-to-one)* – see how they work. Do they need to be shorter – or maybe longer? Keep testing out your affirmations so you get them just right for you. As you say them, you feel them empowering you – motivating you.

Now you need to stand up and find some post-it stickers. I wonder what shape they are – what colour they are. You will also need to find a pen. Pick up the post-it stickers and pen – then walk over to the noticeboard. Remember the affirmations you have created for yourself – just go through them again – say them to yourself *(or out loud)*. Good. Now you need to write them down – one at a time. One affirmation on each post-it sticker.

Think of one of your affirmations – say it to yourself *(or out loud)* – then write it on a post-it sticker. Read and say the affirmation to yourself again *(or out loud)* – then put the post-it sticker on the noticeboard.

Now think of another one of your affirmations – say it to yourself *(or out loud)* – then write it on a post-it sticker. Read and say the affirmation to yourself again *(or out loud)* – then put the post-it sticker on the noticeboard.

Keep going until all your affirmations are on the noticeboard. When you have finished, read each one again. Nod your head when you have finished reading them all again. Well done. Whenever you need to feel motivated – want to remember an affirmation – or add more affirmations to the noticeboard just say to yourself: 'Noticeboard'.

Additional script 5: Recording what you want to say

There are times in everyone's life when it is hard to express your thoughts or feelings. Some people just find it hard to talk in general – they may be shy and not want to talk about themselves. There is absolutely nothing wrong with being a private person. Others do not talk about things because they feel ashamed or embarrassed. They may worry how people are going to react. Others keep things to themselves to protect people – they do not want anyone else to be worried. When people find it difficult express themselves by talking in the conscious state, it is often much easier for them to talk in the trance state – when the subconscious mind is deeply relaxed and does not have a care in the world.

You know that here in the message room there are all sorts of ways to communicate. One method I would like you to try today is recording something you want or need to say – to your baby or *(insert others, e.g. mum; birthing partner; children; doctor; nurse; midwife; relative).*

Find a comfortable place to sit in the message room – a chair or a sofa – somewhere you can relax. Sink down into the seat and breathe nice and slowly.

(Guidance note: the hypnotherapist should decide at this point how they want to proceed – depending what they have planned for the session. Two options are presented below)

Option 1: Talking to baby

Now as you are relaxing more and more – keep breathing nice and steadily – think about some of the things you would like to say to your baby. Maybe you just want to tell him/her how you are feeling today or how you are feeling about the future – how much you are looking forward to their arrival and being in your life. Maybe there are stories you want to tell your baby – things that have happened today, this week or last month. Or stories about the past – your family or friends. Maybe you would like to talk about your hopes and aspirations for the future. I do not know – but you will know what it would be good to tell your baby. What it would be good to share. What would be helpful. What would be reassuring. So just think about that now.

Now I wonder what you want to talk into and record on – a phone, iPad or a Dictaphone. Look around you now and you will see what you need – pick it up in your hand – look at it and then prepare yourself – become familiar with how to start recording, pause and stop the recording whenever you want to. OK – are ready to start recording? Remember you can pause or stop at any time. You can delete and start again. It does not matter how many times you pause, stop or delete. It is all good practice. You can keep recording until it feels right. OK then – ready – press to start recording – and start speaking now. I shall be silent for a few minutes and let you record.

(Guidance note: if working in a group, let there be a fairly long silence – maybe up to two or three minutes. If working with one client, suggest they speak out load so you know what they are recording and then follow up with discussion)

Well done, you have made your first recording. It is safely stored and can be played back any time.

Option 2: Telling someone how you feel

(Guidance note: this option can be used to rehearse something which needs to be said, for example, to a professional or relative when mum/dad is feeling uncomfortable or even dreading doing this. It can be used to work on particular issues, for example, confronting an abuser, rapist etc)

Now just keep relaxing – that's right. I know you have been thinking about *(insert one of the following)*:

- What you want to say to *(insert person)*. It can help to rehearse what you want to say.
- What *(insert person)* did to you. I think it would help you to say what you think and what you feel.

As you are sitting comfortably, feel the strength and confidence that you know is deep inside you. You know you can say what you think in an assertive, not an aggressive way. You just need to be clear.

Imagine now that *(insert person)* is sitting in a chair right opposite you. Look them right in the eye. Before you speak – be clear about what you want to say. Gather your thoughts together. Take your time – do not rush – gather your thoughts. Think about what you need to say.

Now I wonder what you want to talk into and record on – a phone, an iPad or a Dictaphone. Look around you now and you will see what you need – pick it up in your hand – look at it and then prepare yourself – become familiar with how to start recording, pause and stop the recording whenever you want to. OK – are you ready to start recording? Remember you can pause or stop at any time. You can delete and start again. It does not matter how many times you pause, stop or delete. It is all good practice. You can keep recording until it feels right. OK then – ready – press to start recording – and start speaking now. Keep looking at *(person)* sitting in front you. Watch how they react as you record what you want to say to them.

(Guidance note: when the recording has been completed the following questions can be asked)

How did you feel as you were recording what you wanted to say?
How did *(person)* look as you were speaking? *(e.g. facial expression; body language)*
Did *(person)* try to say anything to you?
Do you want to change anything you said – the words or sentences?
Do you want to delete anything?
Do you want to change how you said what you said? *(e.g. loudness; pace of speech; tone)*
Do you want to re-record what you said?

(Guidance note: if another recording is made then use some of the following questions)

How did you feel this time?
How did *(person)* look as you were speaking? *(e.g. facial expression; body language)*

Did *(person)* try to say anything to you?

Do you want to change anything now?

Do you want to change anything you said – the words or sentences?

Do you want to change how you said what you said? *(e.g. loudness; pace of speech; tone)*

Do you want to have another go at recording? Remember it does not matter how many times you pause, stop or delete. Keep going until it feels right.

(Guidance note: the hypnotherapist should work with mum until she is happy with the recording)

Congratulations – you have expressed yourself so well.

Additional script 6: Keeping a journal

Keeping a journal is a lovely way of storing your memories – not just what happened and when – but you can write about how you felt at the time something happened. Reading an entry in a journal can trigger a memory – a thought – a feeling. Lots of exciting things are going to happen to you in the next few weeks and months. It would be lovely to write about events – your thoughts – and your feelings – so you can share the memories with your baby.

Somewhere in the message room there will be shelves or a bookcase and on one shelf you are drawn towards you will find what may look like a book but in fact it is a journal. Find it now. This journal is completely empty at the moment but you are going to put it to good use. Pick up the journal and have a look at it – and in it. I wonder what size it is – what colour the outside is – what colour the pages on the inside are. Feel the outside cover of the journal – feel the pages on the inside.

Find a pen or anything else you would prefer to write with and then go to sit down with your journal. On the front of the journal write: '*(name of mum/dad)*'s Journey'. Let your mind go back to when you first knew you were going to have a baby/become a dad. Just go back in time, slowly recall the memory – the news about the baby. As you drift back – back in time – remember your thoughts and feelings. As you go right back – start to write in your journal – the important memories – thoughts and feelings. Tell me what you are writing in the journal.

(Guidance note: this is a gentle introduction to using the journal and recalling memories. The hypnotherapist can choose to take mum/dad to a specific event/ incident/worry/fear which needs to be worked on. Some general questions/prompts follow)

Tell me what happened then.

Who was there?

What was said?

How did you feel at the time?

Is there anything you would like to read from your journal to the baby?

Is there anything you would like to read from your journal to anyone else?

Is there anything else you need to write in the journal right now?

34 Portfolio of perfect photographs

Introduction

We all carry photographs in our heads. It is said if you see something in your mind's eye, you imagine it and have a clear picture of it in your mind. Our memories can be stored mentally in the subconscious; or physically like in a paper photograph. People who are visual may see a memory in the form of a picture, or a film or a play. People dream in different ways too; some people dream in colour, others in black and white. Therefore, memories and photographs can be stored in all sorts of ways. In the conscious state photographs can be carried with us in various ways too: a paper photograph in a handbag, purse, wallet; on a computer/laptop/iPad; mobile phone and in the cloud.

The purpose of this script is to encourage mum to think about how she wants things to be in the future, to create that image and to strive to achieve perfection. It embeds the idea of having the ability to experiment, make changes and adjustments to get things right.

We must consider that what constitutes a 'family' will be dependent on expectations of society, communities and individuals. In reality, a family can be made up of people who have all kinds of relationships with each other. Often it is not helpful to contemplate what is the norm. A single mum can feel very excluded when people are talking about a traditional family, with two parents and two sets of lovely grandparents. The reality is that many people have been brought up in dysfunctional families and their memories from childhood may not be blissful. Family albums are supposed to show families experiencing happy, memorable events. The hypnotherapist's role is to reassure mum that a family can be made up in different ways – it does not have to be 'traditional' and family members to do not have to be blood-related. Some clients will say their friends are more like their real family than actual family members. This script encourages mum to think about how she wants her family to be through creating a portfolio of photographs.

The script

A professional photographer prepares for a considerable amount of time in order to create the perfect picture. It is not done in a hurry; it is something that is thought about, created through trial and sometimes error, making changes, doing things differently and eventually it is produced. A professional photographer will never just take one photograph. Lots of shots will be taken – click, click, click – maybe from a lot of different angles to see which view is best. The way a professional photographer

DOI: 10.4324/9781003173779-34

takes his shots is a bit like how you are practising self-hypnosis – your breathing – your techniques – working out what is best for you and your baby.

So today imagine you are going to be the professional photographer and you are going to start to create a portfolio of photographs. You are going to create a photograph – how you want things to be for your baby/family. Then in the future you can create more photographs and create a portfolio if you would like to do that. You can create a portfolio of perfect photographs about your pregnancy and the arrival of your baby. Start thinking about some of the important things that are going to happen over the next few months and how you would like things to be. Maybe think about:

- Going for a scan
- Going to a class (hypnobirthing; yoga)
- In the birthing room
- When the baby is born
- When you bring the baby home.

You are going to create some perfect photographs and to do this you need to think, prepare and create. Think, prepare and create. You need to relax your mind really deeply now – go as deep as you can – because the more you relax the more creative your mind will be. Your subconscious mind will work with you to create the perfect photographs.

(Guidance note: if mum is not sure what photographs she might like to take, which could be the case for a very young mum, the hypnotherapist can make some suggestions as follows)

- Going for a scan:
  - different times during the a scan.
  - the actual picture/scan of the baby
- Going to a class (hypnobirthing; yoga):
  - class in action: teacher and participants
  - group photo at end
- In the birthing room:
  - different stages: in between surges
  - pushing
  - caesarean
  - delivery
- When the baby is born:
  - immediately: skin to skin
  - cutting the cord
  - breastfeeding
  - the family
- Bringing baby home:
  - saying 'goodbye' at the hospital
  - arriving home.

What is important to you?
What do you want to happen?
How do you want things to be?

Who is going to be in the photograph?
Where will the photograph be taken? (*e.g. location*)
What is going to be in the photograph? *(e.g. objects)*
Where will you be? *(e.g. standing or sitting)*
What will you be doing? *(e.g. actions/body language)*
What will you be wearing?
What expression will you have on your face?
What will you be feeling inside?
Where will *X* be? *(e.g. standing or sitting)*
What will s/he be doing? *(e.g. actions/body language)*
What will s/he be wearing?
What expression will s/he have on his/her face?

OK – you have set up the scene ready for the photograph – you are ready to take some shots. So, get your camera ready. Look through the lens – see the scene. Make some adjustments if you need to – consider the lighting, the focus – is everything clear to you? Start taking some shots – click, click, click. Make some changes if you need to – move anything – tell the people in the photograph how you want them to look – how you want them to be – how you hope they will feel.

OK – ready – take some more shots – click, click, click. Do you want to make any more changes to the scene you are photographing?

(Guidance note: the hypnotherapist should let mum keep making changes until she is happy with the scene and encourage her to take lots of shots)

Go forward in time – to when you have all the shots you have taken either printed out or right in front of you on a screen. Look at each one – take your time. You are looking for the perfect photograph. As you are looking at each shot you took – when you reject one – ask yourself the reason for that – the reason it was not good enough for your portfolio. Tell me some of the reasons.

Keep going until you find the perfect photograph. You will know when you see it because there will be no need to photoshop this perfect photograph. Tell me when you have chosen it. Describe it to me. How do you feel as you look at this photograph?

Think about what you have done. You thought about what you wanted. You thought about setting the scene. You took some practice runs by taking some shots – click, click, click. You made some changes to get things just right. You took more shots – click, click, click. You created the perfect picture – you had insight. You knew what you wanted to create. You knew what was right for you.

(Guidance note: the hypnotherapist may choose to suggest that mum can take other photographs in this session. However, it can be more effective to leave it to the next session and build the portfolio through the remaining sessions)

Over time you can create a portfolio of photographs. You have created your first photograph today but there will so many more you create in the future. Now you need to decide where will you keep the photographs. They will always be in your mind's eye but where else might you like to store them?

(Guidance note: the hypnotherapist works with mum to store the photographs. Prompts could be: folder; carry case; mobile phone; iPad; computer/laptop)

Congratulations – you have achieved so much today. You have been creative and started your very own portfolio, which you will add to in the future. Think about what you have done. You thought about what you wanted. You thought about setting the scene. You did some practice runs by taking some shots – click, click, click. You made some changes to get things just right. You took more shots – click, click, click. You created the perfect picture – you had insight. You knew what you wanted to create. You knew what was right for you. You have started to create the portfolio of perfect photographs.

Part VII

Working with worries, fears and phobias

35 The old mining village

Introduction

The main purpose of this script is to get rid of anything that is preventing a client from enjoying their pregnancy or is making them anxious about the future birthing, so this could be mum, dad or birthing partner. It could be in relation to a simple concern or worry or something that is more deep-rooted – a fear or phobia or a memory of a past incident/experience. It is important for the hypnotherapist to discuss the issue in the conscious state before using the script in order to explore the client's thoughts, feelings and behaviours associated with the issue. This can be done in more depth once in trance.

The main script takes mum, dad or birthing partner to the old mining village and then there are three additional scripts where fears and memories can be thrown away and emotions released – the churchyard, the well and the pit. The client can choose which place they want to work in. If there are several issues that need to be worked on then it is possible to return to the old mining village in future sessions.

The script

I want to tell you about an old mining village, which nowadays is considered to be a small town. It is curious how things can change, develop and grow. The old mining village was one of several villages in the area whose populations were dependent on the coal industry. Most of the men went down the pit every day of their lives. Sons automatically followed in their fathers' footsteps; it was expected – no choice at all. Today the town has several big roads leading into it. I want you to go back in time and imagine what the old mining village might have looked like many years ago. Imagine that you are walking along a pathway and in the distance, you see a small hump-back bridge – just wide enough for a horse and cart to cross over or in later years one car. Keep walking towards the bridge.

You see a group of men and boys walking in front of you. They are wearing their work clothes. They are chatting away and laughing – looking as though they have not got a care in the world. As you follow behind them towards the bridge you feel a bit different. For some unknown reason you feel like you are going backwards even though you are walking forward. That is because you are going back to visit the old mining village – the way it used to be.

You are still following the group of men and boys. They are going over the bridge now and then they turn off to the right because they need to get to the pit to start their shift. Now you start to cross over the hump-back bridge. You may hear the tinkling of

DOI: 10.4324/9781003173779-35

water which is running under the bridge. Or maybe you hear the splish and splash of some fish as they rise up to the surface of the water. Or the quacking of some ducks, geese or other birds that are around.

Keep going across the bridge and follow the pathway in front of you. You start to see some little houses ahead of you. Some have small gardens at the back. You can see the washing lines – full of clothes. Children are playing out in front of the little houses. Some boys are running about playing chase. Others are throwing and catching a ball. Two girls are holding a skipping rope at each end while two other girls skip in the middle. Women are sitting on their doorsteps chatting away. As you walk by them, they greet you. Stop and chat for a while, if you want to do so.

When you are ready, continue your walk to the heart of the village. I wonder what you will see first. There are lots of places and things to see. Perhaps the village church with its tall spire. The village tavern. The shops – butcher – grocer – the blacksmith who is shoeing horses and ponies. Right in the middle you will see the village green – a place where you can sit and think; relax with your thoughts. Go there now and find somewhere to sit. Sit down and relax.

Imagine that you are sitting with your eyes closed on the village green – feeling really relaxed. I want you think about *(insert issue that has already been discussed in the conscious state)*. Now you need to get rid of that *(issue)* and there are several really good places in the village you could get rid of it forever, so it never troubles you again. There is a churchyard – a well – and a pit where coal is mined. Would you like to go and look at them or do you know already where you would like to get rid of *(issue)*?

(Guidance note: the hypnotherapist can then use one of the additional
scripts below)

Additional script 1: The churchyard

From where you are sitting you should be able to see the spire of the church pointing upwards towards the sky. The church has a graveyard. This might be a really good place to bury *(issue)*. Whilst you are sitting comfortably on the village green – think about *(issue)*. As you are thinking about it tell me what you are thinking about exactly and how that makes you feel.

(Guidance note: the hypnotherapist should leave enough time to explore the issue
in depth. The client may talk about a feeling, fear or previous incident/experience.
Some possible questions/prompts follow below)

Tell me more about this.
Tell me what happened.
Tell me how you feel.
When did this happen?
How long have you felt like this?
When did this start?
How do you feel talking about it now?
What would you like to change/be different?

If you look down onto the grass of the village green you will see there is a big bag right next to your feet. Imagine that you are putting *(issue)* in that bag. Pick up the bag and hold it – it will feel very heavy.

It is time to make your way towards the church now. Take the bag with you – it feels so very heavy. When you reach the church, you will see a gate into the churchyard, which slopes down the hill. Go through the gate and put the bag down on the ground – you can leave it there while you go and have a look around the churchyard. Look for a place where you would like to bury *(issue)*. Tell me when you have found a suitable place. Take your time – there is no need to rush. You will know when you have found the right place. Just tell me when you have found it.

Good. Now look around and somewhere nearby you will find a spade. Now start digging a hole in the ground. Start digging now. Make sure it is big enough and dig the hole really, really deep. Tell me when you have finished. Now go back and pick up the bag – it still feels really heavy. Hold it in your hands and know that it is never going to bother you again. Take the bag to the hole you have dug. In a moment you are going to throw the bag into the hole and you will feel a massive surge of release – a sense of letting go. I am going to count slowly to 5 and when I say 5 throw the bag into the hole – 1, 2, 3, 4, and 5. Throw the bag into the hole. Watch the bag fall slowly and feel that sense of release within you – that freedom. Well done. You know you are never going to feel that very heavy bag again.

Pick up the spade again and fill the hole. As you are filling in the hole acknowledge that *(issue)* has gone forever and you can focus on the future. As you are filling the hole, think about all the good things that are going to happen in the future.

(Guidance: mum/dad/birthing partner is filling the hole the hypnotherapist can embed some positive suggestions/statements)

Additional script 2: The well dressing

You can see the church from where you are sitting on the village green. Just a short distance from the church there is a well. It has been there for hundreds of years. It goes down and down beneath the ground – some say for miles and miles and miles. Every year around the month of June, the villagers dress the well with pictures, which are made of flowers, petals of flowers and leaves – it is a local tradition called 'Well-Dressing'. Can you imagine the top of the well covered in beautiful flowers – all different colours. The well might be a really good place to throw away *(issue)*. Whilst you are sitting comfortably on the village green – think about *(issue)*. As you are thinking about it, tell me what you are thinking about exactly and how that makes you feel.

(Guidance note: the hypnotherapist should leave enough time to explore the issue in depth. Mum/dad/birthing partner may talk about a feeling, fear or previous incident/experience. Some possible questions/prompts follow below)

Tell me more about this.
Tell me what happened.
Tell me how you feel.
When did this happen?
How long have you felt like this?
When did this start?
How do you feel talking about it now?
What would you like to change/be different?

If you look down onto the grass of the village green you will see there is a big bag right next to your feet. Imagine that you are putting *(issue)* in that bag. Pick up the bag and hold it – it will feel very heavy.

It is time to go and find the well – start walking towards the church. Take the bag with you – it feels so very heavy. When you reach the church, you will see the well a short distance away. Go and find it now. Tell me when you get there and put the bag on the ground. Tell me what the well looks like. Look down the well – it is very dark. Can you see anything at all?

It is time to get rid of *(issue)* forever – it will never bother you again. You are going to throw the bag down the well, which is so deep – it goes down for miles and miles and miles. Are you ready? Now go back and pick up the bag – it still feels really heavy. Hold it in your hands and know that it is never going to bother you again. In a moment you are going to throw the bag into the well and as the bag travels down and down the deep well – travelling all those miles and miles and miles – you will feel a massive surge of release – a sense of letting go. I am going to count slowly to *5* and when I say *5* throw the bag down the well – *1, 2, 3, 4,* and *5*. Throw the bag into the well now. See the bag falling and feel that sense of release within you – that freedom. Well done. You know you are never going to feel that very heavy bag again.

Now it is time to dress the well with a picture. A picture of how you want things to be in the future. Think about the future while you are searching for some flowers, petals and leaves so you can make your own well dressing picture – a picture of how you want things to be.

(Guidance: the hypnotherapist should work with mum/dad/birthing partner to dress the well. Discussing in depth his/her hopes and aspirations for the future and embedding some positive suggestions/statements)

Additional script 3: The pit

The pit is where the miners dig for coal. They spend hours and hours beneath the earth – in the dark with only candles as light. They have pit ponies to help them bring the coal back up to the surface. It's holiday time and the pit is closed for 2 weeks, so this would be a really good time to get rid of *(issue)*. Whilst you are sitting comfortably on the village green – think about *(issue)*. As you are thinking about it, tell me what you are thinking about exactly and how that makes you feel.

(Guidance note: the hypnotherapist should leave enough time to explore the issue in depth. Mum/dad/birthing partner may talk about a feeling, fear or previous incident/experience. Some possible questions/prompts follow below)

Tell me more about this.
Tell me what happened.
Tell me how you feel.
When did this happen?
How long have you felt like this?
When did this start?
How do you feel talking about it now?
What would you like to change/be different?

Even though the pit is closed the entrance is always open. If you look down onto the grass of the village green you will see there is a big bag right next to your feet. Imagine that you are putting *(issue)* in that bag. Pick up the bag and hold it – it will feel very heavy. It is time to go and find the pit, which is located just outside of the village. You need to go back the way you came – back towards the hump-back bridge. Take the bag with you – it feels so very heavy. When you see the bridge in front of you take the road to the left and that will lead you to the pit entrance. You will see buildings and structures standing on the land – the pithead is where you can get down into the pit. Walk towards the pithead when you see it. Tell me when you get there.

There is a shaft that goes down from the pithead into the pit. There is a gate that leads you onto a platform which will take you down into the pit. Step onto the platform and as you do that you are aware of how heavy the bag is that you have been carrying. Close the gate and the platform starts to move down and down and down. As you are moving down you feel the bag you are holding is getting lighter. As you travel down and down, darkness surrounds you but strangely you are feeling lighter and lighter. The darkness makes you feel safe and protected. When the platform comes to a standstill you see the face of a pony looking at you. The pony is going to show you the way – the way to the coal face. Just follow the pony and as you walk the bag feels lighter. Keep following the pony.

When the pony stops you realise it is because he is too big to go any further. He looks at you and nods his head. You know you need to get down on the floor and crawl forward. Drag the bag with you and crawl until you cannot go any further – until you get to a dead end. You will see a wall made of coal – you have reached the coalface. Lift the bag and place it at the coalface. Look around you – see if you can find any coal, rocks or anything else to cover the bag, so you cannot see it anymore. *(Issue)* will never bother you again.

Now crawl back to find the pony. As you are crawling you feel free – feel the lightness within you – you are happy and optimistic. You can look forward to the future. Keep crawling forward. You see the pony that will lead you forward and back to the platform. Now you and the pony are travelling upwards on the platform – upwards to the open air and to the future.

(Guidance note: the hypnotherapist will embed positive suggestions/statements as mum/dad/birthing partner returns to the pithead and open air)

36 Ice sculpture

Introduction

I wrote this script originally to deal with any fear mum, dad or birthing partner might have had for a while (even since childhood, adolescence or earlier in adulthood) which could have some negative impact on the pregnancy or birth. A good example and a common fear, which is extremely hard to admit, is dad fearing he is going to pass out at the sight of all the blood during the birthing. The script can be used for any fear or phobia and it is advisable to book a separate individual session to work with this. In some cases, more than one session might be needed. Although the script was written for long-established fears, I also use it for any new fears which develop during a pregnancy. For example, if mum has miscarried or had a stillbirth before, she may fear that she is going to lose this baby as well.

The script

You have told me about your fear of *(insert)*. Well, it has been bothering you for long enough – now is the time to get rid of it forever. As you work on this you may feel uncomfortable but I want you to try to stay with it as long as you can. I am saying this now because I want you to think about the last time you were thinking about *(fear)*.

I know this is not very pleasant for you but go back in time and think about how you were feeling the last time you were thinking or experiencing *(fear)*. Just drift back – let your mind remember – slowly drift back. Let the thoughts and feelings return. Tell me where you are and what is happening.

> *(Guidance note: the hypnotherapist needs to get as much information as possible from mum/dad/birthing partner about what s/he is thinking about; the following prompts can be used if required)*

Where are you?
What are you doing?
What are you thinking?
How are you feeling?
How are you feeling now as you are experiencing it again?
Is anything happening to your body as you are feeling this? *(e.g. sweaty palms; shaking; palpitations)*

> *(Guidance note: the hypnotherapist may want mum/dad/birthing partner to remember several times when s/he has been thinking about or experiencing the fear – in order to get more information about it)*

DOI: 10.4324/9781003173779-36

Well done for thinking about *(fear)*. Now it is time to get rid of it forever. I want you to imagine that you are in the kitchen of a hotel. The kitchen is currently closed – there is no-one else around. In this hotel they organise lots of important functions and one of the things they are really good at is making ice sculptures. There are several freezers in the kitchen and if you look in any of them you will find many blocks of uncut ice.

Perhaps now you would like to find one of the function rooms. As you go into the room, you notice everything has been set out for a function which is going to take place very soon. You will see chairs, tables for people to sit at and banqueting tables where food will be set out. You also see all sorts of decorations on the tables and around the room. Now as you are walking around having a look at everything, I want you to start thinking about *(fear)* again. Just stay with it as before.

In a moment you are going to turn around and look at one of the large banqueting tables which is in the room. Keeping thinking about *(fear)*. On the count of *3* – you will turn around and see *(fear)* in the shape of an ice sculpture. *1, 2,* and *3* – turn around. See *(fear)* in the shape of an ice sculpture on the banqueting table.

What does the ice sculpture look like? *(note: it may present as an object or a person)*
Describe it to me.
How are you feeling as you look at the ice sculpture?
Is there anything you want to say to the ice sculpture?

Now it is time for the ice sculpture to melt. You are going to make the ice sculpture melt very quickly – it is not going to be a long thawing out. It is going to melt quickly – very quickly indeed. You may want to turn up the heating in the function room. Make it really hot. Find the thermostat in the function room and turn it up as high as it will go. You can also bring anything into the function room to help you melt the ice sculpture. Is there anything you need? Now make the ice sculpture melt.

See the top of the ice sculpture start to melt. See the top of it starting to disappear. The ice is turning to water – running down the rest of the sculpture. The ice continues to melt. The *(fear)* is going away – feel it melting away – not existing anymore. Feel *(fear)* losing its strength. It is melting, melting away – part by part. Feel *(fear)* melting away – it no longer exists.

> *(Guidance note: the hypnotherapist then needs to encourage mum/dad/birthing partner to keep working on melting the rest of the ice sculpture. Depending on what the ice sculpture is the hypnotherapist should aim to talk through each part as it is melting away and then repeat the following after each part has disappeared)*

Look now at *(next part of the ice sculpture)* start to melt. See the *(next part of the ice sculpture)* start to melt. See it starting to disappear. The ice is turning to water – running down the rest of the ice sculpture. The ice continues to melt. The *(fear)* is going away – feel it melting away – not existing anymore. Feel *(fear)* losing its strength. It is melting, melting away. Feel *(fear)* melting away.

There is hardly anything left of the ice sculpture – just one little bit is left. So watch the last bit melt away. The ice has all gone – it exists no more. All that is left now is a pool of water. You need to throw it away. So how are you going to get rid of that pool of water? Do that now.

Well done. You have melted the whole ice sculpture. *(Fear)* no longer exists. Welcome that feeling of freedom from fear. It will never bother you again.

> *(Guidance note: the hypnotherapist should then embed positive suggestions to replace the fear)*

37 The book of untruths

Introduction

A first pregnancy mum-to-be may worry about whether she is capable of getting through a pregnancy, giving birth and eventually being a good mum. The doubt and lack of confidence may seem a huge problem to that mum, but other pregnant mums may also be lacking confidence for a variety of very different reasons. Maybe they had problems in a previous pregnancy or during birth and they feel they failed in some way; or they do not believe they are a very good parent – they could be doubting and questioning themselves on a regular basis.

People can lack confidence because of what has been said to them in the past. Something someone has said may remain suppressed in the subconscious mind for a long time or if it is something which was said regularly, the person can come to believe it is true. For example, in my work with survivors of abuse I hear frequently how the perpetrator of abuse has told the victim they are 'stupid', 'useless' or 'worthless'. Victims of bullying have often been tormented by things said about how they look. Mum or dad may have a history of abuse or bullying, which has resulted in low self-esteem and lack of confidence and this in turn may affect how they are going to deal with pregnancy, birthing and parenthood. Hypnotherapy could be needed to build confidence. Ego boosting is always very useful to address this (see scripts in Part X), but in my own practice as a hypnotherapist I like to go back to find the root cause of the problem and deal with that in the first instance. This was my reason for writing the script below, which can be used for mum or dad.

The script can be used to help mum get rid of any negative beliefs she has about herself which have been affecting her for some time – before she was pregnant (even back to childhood). It can be used to build self-belief and confidence. Alternatively, the script can be used solely to focus on any old wives' tales or stories mum has been told, which are very unhelpful. Within the script there are also elements of promoting some assertiveness techniques. Some people can become very ego-centric and regale mum with stories about their own experiences, not taking into account what effect this might be having on mum. If a person has a tendency to talk a lot (especially about themselves) then mum needs to be able to stop the unwanted chatter assertively.

The script

The subconscious mind is always ready to listen. It listens. It watches. It learns. It accumulates information. It stores information. That is how your subconscious mind

DOI: 10.4324/9781003173779-37

knows everything about you and knows the reasons for you being as you are. It understands the way you think – feel – and behave.

What I would like you to think about now are the things you have been told since the moment you were born; and the fact that maybe some of those things were not true. You may have been told some untruths without any harm really being intended. In fact, some of the untruths may have been well meant. Like when you were a child, you may have been told if you were good all year round then Father Christmas would bring the presents you wanted. Or when a tooth fell out if you put it under your pillow the tooth fairy would replace the tooth with some money. Well, you know now that neither Father Christmas nor the tooth fairy exist. You probably remember other things that you might have believed at the time: 'If you eat lots of carrots you'll see better in the dark'. No malice or harm was intended and I want you to remember that. Sometimes people say things with the best intentions.

(Guidance note: if the hypnotherapist is working with someone who has been abused or bullied insert the following paragraph before proceeding:

However, there are some people who deliberately say things to hurt you. They know exactly what word or phrase will you hurt you – and they say it over and over and over again. They say it so often you may come to believe it to be true. That is just not right and I want you to remember that. Some people tell untruths and you must not believe them – or if you have to come believe them you have to unlearn the untruths)

What I would also like you to give some consideration to is that some people have a tendency to exaggerate. Or the more a person tells a tale, they embellish it and it becomes more detailed – maybe further from the truth. They believe it did happen just as they are telling the tale in the here and now.

When you are pregnant, many people are going to tell you about their own experiences. Some people may be very helpful but others might tell you things that make you feel anxious, worried or create some fear. If that happens, remember you have the right to stop them right there and tell them you do not want to hear any more. I know you are a very polite person and would not want to offend anyone but you can express your wishes assertively without being aggressive. You just have to be honest and tell them three things. Firstly, that you have heard what they have said. Secondly, how it has made you feel. Thirdly, what you want them to do – that is you do not want to hear any more. Being assertive is not being rude – you have the right to say what you want to happen.

So, let's think about some of the things that you might have heard or been told that maybe are not true or helpful. I want you to imagine that you are holding a book in your hand. The title of the book is 'The book of untruths' by *(insert mum's name)*. I am wondering what the book looks like.

Is it a hardback or paperback?
How big is it?
What colour is the title written in?
What colour is your name written in?
Is there anything written or drawn on the front cover?

Now open the book and look at the title page: 'The book of untruths' by *(insert mum's name)*. Feel the paper. Smell the pages. When you are ready, I want you to start flicking through the pages. On a page there will be an untruth that you have been told some-where in your lifetime. You will see the first few chapters are about your early life and the later chapters focus on your adulthood and recent times. Just take your time – start flicking through.

Some of the untruths do not really matter as they have not affected you at all. How-ever, some of the untruths have affected you in unhelpful ways – they have not bene-fited you at all. Some of them may have played on your mind. You may have heard an inner voice telling you the untruth again and again. Maybe you did not believe it at first but, the more you thought about it, you convinced yourself it was true.

So, when you feel ready to stop flicking through the book, let the book of untruths just fall open at one page.

(Guidance note: the hypnotherapist should then encourage mum to remember more about the untruth and talk about it. Some prompts are included in the next part of the script)

What untruth is written on the page?
Who said that to you?
When was that?
Who was there?
What was happening at the time?
How did you feel at the time this was said?
How do you feel about it now?
What is the real truth?

(Guidance note: the hypnotherapist should embed the truth and use some positive ego strengthening)

OK, now open the book at another page.

(Guidance note: the hypnotherapist repeats the process/questions. It is up to the hypnotherapist how many untruths they want to address in a session. In some cases, there may only be one or even two untruths written in the book. In others, there may be many)

Now you have explained to me that you have been told some things since you became pregnant that have worried you *(insert as appropriate)*. Go to the very back of the book where you will see the latest untruths you have been told. Just relax – and very slowly start flicking through the book – going towards the front. You need to find the untruth (or untruths) that caused this worry. Tell me when you have found the right page and look at the untruth you have been told.

What untruth is written on the page?
Who said that to you?
When was that?
Who was there?
What was happening at the time?
How did you feel at the time this was said?
How do you feel about it now?
What is the real truth?

(Guidance note: the hypnotherapist should embed the truth and use some positive ego strengthening)

Good. You now know and accept that all these untruths you have been told are totally not true – they serve no purpose in your life at all. They have not benefited you in any way whatsoever. It is time to get rid of them once and for all. So how would you like to do that? What do you want to do with the pages and the book?

(Guidance note: the hypnotherapist follows mum's lead on this and works with her to get rid of the pages and book)

Well done. So now I want you to start writing your own book: 'The book of truths' by *(insert mum's name).* Find yourself a book you would like to write in. You will need a pen as well. It would be good if you could start the book now with some of the truths you have learnt about yourself. Do that now. Now write the truths about your baby – your pregnancy. Do that now. Think about them now – the truths – and as you write each one in the book – tell me what you have written.

You have told me that some people *(mention specific people if possible)* have been telling you things *(insert specifics if possible)*, which have not been helpful. I want you to start thinking about phrases you can use to stop them in the future so you do not have to listen anymore. Take your time and then tell me what you might say to *(name of person/people)*.

(Guidance note: mum should be encouraged to use her own response/language and experiment by saying them out loud, that is, rehearse them and change them if needs be. The following can be used as prompts/suggestions and mum can change to use her preferred words/language style)

I don't believe that is correct.
I know that will not happen to me and my baby.
I don't accept that at all.
That is not true.
What you are saying is not helping me.
I'd prefer it if you didn't keep telling me/talking about this.
I don't want to have this conversation.
I don't want to hear any negative thoughts.
I don't want to hear any more stories/tales.

That is really good. Keep saying it out loud and then write it in your book of truths. You have come up with some really good responses.

Now through the rest of your pregnancy it will be helpful when you come back into trance to write more truths in your book. You could write your affirmations and mantras in there too – because they are truths.

Part VIII

Dealing with trauma and the unexpected

38 It is your body

Introduction

Nowadays there is a lot of emphasis on body image. Sometimes too much importance is placed upon it and the need for perfection. There could be all sorts of reasons for a person not liking their body or people looking at them. Some people feel embarrassed about or ashamed of their body; this could be because of having:

- Received derogatory comments about their body/how they look
- Current/past injuries (e.g. cuts, bruises, burn marks)
- Had surgery
- Transitioned
- Lost a limb
- Scars
- A disability
- Been abused (physically and/or sexually).

The problem may not just relate to the body being looked at; it can also be connected to being touched in any way. So, having to undergo any sort of medical examination can be very traumatic for some mums. I have worked with a lot of women who are constantly reminded about the physical harm which has been inflicted upon them because of the physical damage which still causes them pain (e.g. internal damage which causes pain when having sex). There are many scripts in the book which will help mum to distract herself by using hypnosis when she is going through a procedure (even a simple one like having a scan), but the script below aims to get mum to think specifically about her own body, how it functions and to promote positivity. In addition, it can be very effective to use this script when developing a birthing plan (see Chapter 27).

The script

I want you to think about your body. Your body – that is carrying your baby. Your own body which grew from being an egg to a foetus – to being a small body when you were born and then it has grown through childhood, adolescence and into adulthood. It is growing again now with the baby inside you. Your body has lots happening within it. Just think about – your skeleton – and the muscles and skin holding it all together – and all the organs inside your body working away. When you think about it,

DOI: 10.4324/9781003173779-38

your body does a great job. It is your very own body and you can make choices about what happens to it from now on and into the future.

I know that in the past your body has been harmed – violated – invaded *(or insert any other trauma)*. It is only natural that what has happened to you in the past and what has been done to your body is going to affect how you feel and how you react to certain situations. It is only natural to experience different emotions – maybe sadness, shame, anger or fear *(insert any other emotion mum has talked about)*. I know you are worried about *(insert as appropriate)*:

- being in hospital
- the procedures that might have to be carried out
- your body being looked at/touched/examined.

Remember, this is your body and you have the right to say what you want to happen or what you do not want to happen. You have the right to make your wishes known. People need permission from you before they do anything to your body.

You have been through a lot in the past. Since then, you have gained strength – you have taken control – and that is what you can do when something has to be done to your body during your pregnancy or when you are birthing. You can ask questions. You can say what you want to happen and what you do not want to happen. You have the confidence to speak out and say what you want to happen.

Remember that the professionals around you are there to help you and your baby. They want to see your baby arrive safely into the world. It is their job to do the best for you and your baby, but in order to do so you need to speak with them – tell them how you feel – what you want to happen. You need to trust the people who are going to help your baby come into the world.

Celebrate your body and the great job it is doing. It conceived your baby. It is helping your baby to grow. It will help your baby start his/her journey into world. It will bring your baby safely and easily into the world. It is your body – be proud of it – and the great job it is doing.

39 Distraction

Introduction

One of the main objectives for any hypnotherapist is to create and work with positivity. It is important to get the client to have positive thoughts and get away from any negative thoughts they may have. Some clients can initially present with a negative attitude, have a pessimistic view of life or may always consider what may be the worst outcome. Any negativity needs to be worked on as early as possible in order to create a more positive attitude and for the hypnotherapy to proceed. Professionals who regularly assess risk and undertake risk assessments in the jobs they do are always considering the dangers, that is, the worst possible outcomes. I am not suggesting a hypnotherapist should introduce the word 'danger' or create fear for a pregnant mum or couple by discussing all the things that might go wrong during pregnancy or birthing. However, the reality is that sometimes the unexpected can happen and it can be helpful to have done some preparation beforehand – although one cannot prepare for every eventuality.

The reality is that mum could have to undergo some procedure, which she did not envisage happening or she may talk about having a specific a fear, such as:

- Use of forceps
- Having stitches
- Having a caesarean section.

Other mums may have specific fears related to what has happened to them in the past and consequently they do not like being touched at all and any medical examination is going to be traumatic for them (this is a particular issue for victims of sexual abuse). Specific work needs to be undertaken for these situations. The purpose of the script below is to reinforce the fact that hypnosis can be used as a distraction and to reinforce what has been learnt already. Therefore, it should be used towards the end of the planned group classes or individual sessions. It is also useful for dad/birthing partner to type out part of the script so s/he can read it out in case of an unexpected event occurring during the birthing. Dad/birthing partner needs to practise delivery of the script (reading slowly, their tone, pitch, etc.), which should have been a subject taught in classes/sessions.

Two very short additional scripts are included after the main script, which can be used in the event of the unexpected happening. I give these to dad/birthing partner as handouts in case they are needed during birthing.

DOI: 10.4324/9781003173779-39

The script

Close your eyes and start relaxing in the way you enjoy most. Just breathe steadily and start going into trance, which you can do so well now. You have learnt so many things during the past few weeks/months – and that is what I want you to think about in today's session. You understand how your subconscious mind is there to protect you. You also know that your subconscious mind remembers everything you have ever seen, heard or learnt. You also know how powerful your subconscious mind is and you can face any situation and deal with it in a positive way. You know that practising self-hypnosis benefits you and going into trance can distract you – take you away from things. You have learnt so many new things since coming here and have so many techniques to help you with your pregnancy and birthing. You can breathe so well. You have your safe place *(insert any other specific technique already learnt for distraction)*. You can travel in your mind anyway you want – to anywhere you want to go.

Today I want you to think about a new way of travelling in your mind so that, if you need to do so, you can take yourself away from your physical body when something might be happening to it or something is being done to it which is uncomfortable for you. Now it is up to you how you travel to get away. I wonder if you might like to travel slowly and gently or whether you prefer to travel at great speed. Think about travelling slowly first. Just imagine that a big bubble is in front of you. You can see into the bubble which is completely empty. Just touch the outside of the bubble and feel how soft it is. Now walk through that soft layer and walk into the bubble. Now feel the inside wall of the bubble – it is very hard – it is there to protect to you. Now try to look through the wall of the bubble – it is turning misty and the bubble starts to move. You can tell the bubble to go in any direction you want it to – just start moving now – slowly and gently. You feel safe and protected inside the bubble – moving away.

Now think about moving at great speed. Imagine a Formula 1 racing car. I wonder what colour it is and whether it has got a number or any names written on the sides of it. You are going to drive the fast racing car. You are wearing all the protective clothing a racing driver needs – helmet, bodysuit, gloves and boots. Get into the car. Put on your seat belt. Start the engine – rev it up – hear and feel how powerful the engine is. Put the car into gear and off you go. Wow – how fast the car is going in just a couple of seconds. You are whizzing around the racing track. Drive around the track a few times – enjoy the speed of it all. Then find an exit and drive the car anywhere you want to go. Feel that speed – leaving everything else behind.

So now you are travelling – anyway you want – slow or fast. Travelling away from whatever you need to get away from. The journey you are taking is distracting you – taking you away – you are becoming distracted. You are distracted from the past – you are distracted from any negative thoughts, feelings or actions. Nothing is going to intrude on your positivity. You are enjoying the journey you are taking now. You are thinking positive thoughts. You know you can achieve anything you want to do. So, as you are travelling now – think about the positive things you have to look forward to in the future.

(Guidance note: the hypnotherapist needs to get mum to be very specific about the immediate future and the weeks ahead. It is important that the positives are written down so dad/birthing partner can use them in the script s/he may use/read out in an emergency situation)

I want you to tell me about the things you are looking forward to.
One by one visualise each thing you are looking forward to.
Explain to me what are you looking forward to exactly.
How do you think you will feel?
Experience that feeling now.

(Guidance note: so when the script is written out for dad/birthing partner the
following will be inserted:

So while you are travelling remember all the things you are looking forward to:

1.
2.
3.
4.
5.
6.

Now think about each one. Visualise [number 1]
Tell me what is happening
Tell me how you are feeling
Visualise [number 2]
Dad/birthing partner continues through the list.

The hypnotherapist or dad/birthing partner can also use some of these positive
commands:

- *You understand how self-hypnosis works*
- *You can self-hypnotise*
- *You can distract yourself*
- *You know what to do*
- *You know hypnosis works*
- *You have practised so hard*
- *You can go to wonderful places*
- *Leave the conscious state now*
- *Go into trance now*
- *You will not feel pain*
- *Imagine – imagine – imagine*
- *Focus on…*
- *Bring your attention to…*
- *You can do this*
- *You will do this*
- *Believe in yourself)*

Additional script 1: Dealing with the unexpected

Things can happen when you least expect it. You know life can throw things at you
and it may seem very unfair. In those situations, you might feel you have not got the

strength to cope. You feel like giving up. I know you are feeling tired right now – you feel like you have no energy left. You just want everything to be over and done with. I want you to remember the strength that you have deep within you. It really is not very long now until your baby is going to come into the world. I know this is not what you wanted – not how you wanted things to be, but you can face and deal with the unexpected – yes you can.

Additional script 2: The wall

Sometimes it is good to get away from things. I am not suggesting that you run away or hide from things – rather it can be helpful to put something in between you and whatever is going on. Putting something in between you can stop you thinking about what is happening. So, I want you to imagine that you are going to build a wall. You are going to build a wall to stop you thinking about *(insert procedure)*. A wall can be made of different materials – bricks – stones – concrete – timber. You choose what you want your wall to be made of and then start building it. Build your wall so it is very wide but it is also very high. Do that now. Make that wall strong and impenetrable. Tell me when you have finished. Look at the wall see how high and strong it is. By looking at that wall you stop thinking about *(insert procedure)*. The wall can stop all intrusive thoughts. Look deep into the wall. The wall makes you feel safe.

40 The shadow

Introduction

I originally wrote 'The shadow' for clients who had experienced some form of abuse. When survivors of abuse first come for therapy they often believe they will never be able to leave the past behind. I know I say frequently: 'You cannot change what has happened in the past but you can change the way you think about it'. That is what hypnotherapy is about – facing and dealing with what has happened and planning for the future. What survivors find unhelpful is being told: 'It's time to move on'. I try to avoid using the term 'moving on', as it can be very irritating. There are scripts in this book which use regression techniques to relive events and incidents in order to release the emotions attached. Using 'The shadow' is an alternative way of letting go of what has been hindering a client.

The script

You are standing very still on a pavement. It is a bright sunny day – not a cloud in the sky. You can feel the sun beating down on the pavement. The pavement is next to a road. The road is very busy – lots of traffic – cars – vans – lorries – motorbikes – bicycles. It is very noisy. The pavement you are standing on is very clear – clear of people. You are standing very still – you have turned away from the road. You are looking straight in front of you.

As you are looking in front of you, I want you to start thinking about the past – what has been troubling you – what you have been dragging with you into the present *(insert specifics if appropriate, e.g. types of abuse, harm or a specific traumatic event)*. I know it feels uncomfortable but stay with your memories for a short while – remember what has happened to you – what has been done to you – what has been said to you.

Stay standing very still, but now turn your head around – maybe twist your body slightly so you can look behind you. Look behind you and then down onto the pavement. You see a shadow. Not a shadow of yourself but a shadow. Look how dark the shadow is. Look at the shape of the shadow. In that shadow see all the things that have happened to you – the things that have been done to you – the things that have been said to you. In the shadow see everything that you have been carrying with you – everything you have been dragging with you into the present.

A shadow is dark. A shadow makes its presence known – it feels like it is always there. It follows you about – it can make you feel like you can never shake it off or get away from it. It sticks to you like glue. It can make you feel like you are stuck – you cannot

DOI: 10.4324/9781003173779-40

move forward. It can make you feel like you are suffocating. There is no escape. It can make you feel like you are being followed and you need to watch every step you take. It can make you constantly look over your shoulder. The shadow is haunting you – day and night. A shadow is dark – it feels like it is always there – there is no escape.

Look again at the shadow that is behind you now. It is time to get rid of it. It is time to leave the shadow behind. This shadow has been following you around for far too long. You know your subconscious mind is a very powerful thing and that it will help you achieve anything you really want to do. You do not want this shadow in your life any longer. You do not want this shadow following you around. It is time that you get rid of it. It is time to leave the shadow behind. You want to live your life in brightness not darkness.

So take one last look at the shadow which is behind you. You know the time has come to leave the shadow behind. You know you have the strength to leave it behind. In the past you may have felt that you could never shake it off – or run away from it – you could never get rid of it – it would always be with you. You feel differently now. You know the time is right. You know you have the strength to leave the shadow and darkness behind – forever.

Look at the shadow. Is there anything you want to say to it before you leave it behind?

(Guidance note: the hypnotherapist should wait for a response and,
if something needs to be said, allow time to work with this)

Now is the time to say 'goodbye' to the shadow. You are taking control. Tell the shadow to stay where it is. Tell the shadow not to move. Tell the shadow not to follow you. Do that now. Feel the strength deep within you as you are taking control – telling the shadow it can no longer follow you. And once again – tell the shadow to stay where it is. Tell the shadow not to move. Tell the shadow not to follow you. Now you are ready to move away from the shadow – leave it behind forever. You are ready to do this. You are feeling strong – empowered – excited.

On the count of *3* you are going to walk away confidently – leaving the shadow behind. Ready – you can do this – *1*, *2*, and *3*. Walk away now. Do not look back. Walk at a pace that is good for you. Feel confident – strong – empowered– excited. You are walking away from the shadow and the darkness. You are walking into brightness – the future. As you stride forward become aware of the future – sense new beginnings. Think about what you want to do – what you want to achieve – and you will do it. Nothing is holding you back – keep walking forward and feel that sense of freedom and the excitement that comes with it. Walk a little quicker now – get to your future more quickly. Enjoy the freedom and excitement – think about the future. Look at the brightness in front of you. What do you see?

(Guidance note: the hypnotherapist can choose to work on the future
and set specific aims and objectives)

Part IX

Loss and bereavement

41 Loss and bereavement

One of the major issues that can come up when working with mums and dads/birthing partners is loss and bereavement. This is one of the main reasons I wanted to write this book. As I said right at the beginning, hypnotherapists may need to use their skills and expertise which other people running hypnobirthing groups may not have. Being pregnant or being a birthing partner can trigger all sorts of memories and losses. It is a well-known fact that grief cannot fit into a specific timescale. A loss can have been experienced decades ago and then something triggers some aspect of that loss and the floodgates open; a person can literally weep like the loss has only just happened. This is why older women in their 80s or 90s can still grieve for babies they miscarried or lost in other ways when they were in their teens or 20s.

Hypnotherapists may already have specific ways of working with loss and bereavement and may favour certain scripts, which can also be used when working with pregnancy and birthing. In this chapter I want to highlight some of the losses a hypnotherapist may have to work with when dealing with pregnancy and birthing. If a hypnotherapist wishes to learn more about loss and bereavement, I would suggest they read some of the traditional, well-established texts written by Elizabeth Kubler-Ross[1] and Colin Murray Parkes[2] as well as the later texts by those authors.[3]

I have found in my own practice that on occasions I have been working with individual clients and it suddenly becomes apparent that they have a common issue. When this happens, it can be beneficial to set up a group to bring those clients together and work on that particular issue. Loss and bereavement is a phrase which covers many aspects of grief. In a group, grief therapy can be used but it is possible for that group to be more focussed and concentrate on a more specific loss, such as discussed below.

The past and keeping secrets

I have worked with a significant number of clients over the years who have kept information about their past and significant events to themselves – often for very good and justifiable reasons. A pregnancy can trigger all sorts of questions and doubts about whether information about the past should be shared now, but also in relation to whether something should be done about unresolved issues before the baby arrives. Typical 'secrets' or dilemmas a client may have can be in relation to previous abortion, pregnancy, adoption, history of abuse – things they have never shared with their partner or anyone else. The hypnotherapist needs to be careful about confidentiality issues and give clear explanations (more than once) especially when working with couples, who may engage in individual sessions. Each client needs to give consent about

DOI: 10.4324/9781003173779-41

what can and cannot be shared with their partner. This is why I always get a mum and birthing partner to sign separate consent forms and explain that anything said in an individual session is confidential to that person – there should be no expectation of 'sharing'.

Miscarriage/stillbirth

When thinking about loss and bereavement in relation to pregnancy and birthing, a woman who has experienced a miscarriage or a stillbirth may immediately spring to mind. As discussed in other chapters, the hypnotherapist must not just focus on work to be undertaken with mum, a dad/birthing partner could have been greatly affected by such a loss as well. Thought needs to be given to dads, siblings, grandparents and possibly other relatives, who could also have been affected by a loss and consequently may be experiencing anxiety about the current pregnancy. The subject of 'fear' will need more consideration. One of the most common fears is that that history is going to repeat itself. Another fear is that it will be impossible ever to have a baby at all.

If a mum has experienced a miscarriage and/or stillbirth, hopefully she will disclose this during the initial assessment. It is important to discuss this thoroughly in order to ascertain whether mum has accepted and worked through the loss. It can be helpful to know whether she had any formal counselling or therapy at the time or whether it is needed now. If mum is still grieving, it can be beneficial to work on this at the outset in order to reduce any stress, fears and anxiety which otherwise might affect the pregnancy. Also, it needs to be emphasised again that a birthing partner might need separate sessions to work on their experience of loss.

The hypnotherapist also needs to be mindful of anniversary blues. Women who miscarry can remember and grieve on the day the baby was lost or on the date the baby was due. If the current baby is due around either of these dates, this can trigger feelings of loss and grief early in or throughout the pregnancy.

Deaths

The subconscious is there to protect a person; it will work in a way it believes is best. It can be a normal occurrence for a person in the conscious state not to understand why they are thinking, feeling and behaving in a certain way. How many times does a thought pop into your head and you wonder why it has when it is something that you have not thought about in ages? In another situation you might suddenly burst into tears, feel overwhelmed but have no idea why – but something you have subconsciously seen or heard will have triggered a memory. Being pregnant can trigger the memory of losing someone (child or adult) which happened a long time ago. It can become clear to the hypnotherapist that a session focusing on that loss is needed. If a death (or more than one death) is discussed, it is useful to get information about dates. Sometimes the baby in the current pregnancy is expected to be born around the date of the death.

Not knowing a parent

Another pertinent issue could be that mum or dad/birthing partner never knew one or both of their parents. Maybe they think they have accepted this fact, but the pregnancy could trigger all sorts of thoughts about the meaning of family and the family/parent they never had. Consequently, doubts and questions could arise and maybe the need to find out about a parent or actually find them.

Adoption

There are two things to consider in regard to adoption. Firstly, mum may have had a previous pregnancy and given up her baby for adoption; this could have affected mum and also dad if he was aware of this. Secondly, mum or her birthing partner may have been adopted themselves. As mentioned above, this could bring up all sorts of emotions and possible dilemmas about finding a birth parent(s).

Knowing that a child will be taken into care

For some mums, they know they are going to experience the loss of the baby they are carrying because a decision has already been taken that the baby will be taken into care. This decision will not have been taken lightly. A pre-birth assessment will have been undertaken by a social worker and maybe other professionals/workers; and mum has probably attended safeguarding meetings. A hypnotherapist could have a vital part to play in providing therapy to help mum accept that the baby is going to be taken from her and would have to be part of any safeguarding/protection plan which is developed (either for the baby or mum). The hypnotherapist may also be asked to attend safeguarding meetings to plan for the work to be undertaken with mum.

There could be many different aspects to the work that may be required. The decision to take a baby into care does not necessarily mean that mum will never get care of the baby in the future. There may be the expectation that mum needs to develop parenting skills which will be undertaken by other professionals, A hypnotherapist could be involved in dealing with the initial loss of having to hand over the baby but there could also be issues relating to mum's past, such as, abuse, anger issues, drug or alcohol misuse/dependency. When working with such issues, there could be a need for therapy to work on lack of self-confidence and/or low self-esteem.

Loss through separation or divorce

It is more common nowadays for couples to separate and divorce, which again can make life complicated when children are involved. Some parents do not see children from a previous relationship. Those children are going to have a new sibling and decisions may need to be made about contact and introducing the new baby. In my own practice, I have mainly provided support for male clients who have lost contact with their children because a relationship has ended – through separating or going through a divorce. Of course, women can also lose contact. In some cases, access can be denied by law, but more commonly loss of contact can happen gradually. The feelings of regret or guilt can be presented and are issues to be worked on.

Surrogacy

Surrogates are rarely mentioned in hypnobirthing texts, yet they are playing a vital role in helping the intended parents. A surrogate will need help in the practical sense regarding pregnancy and birthing just like any other pregnant woman, but she might also require an individual session to prepare her for a different kind of loss. Most surrogates will not have taken on the role of lightly. They will have given it a great deal of thought and hopefully had in-depth discussions with the intended parents before committing to the role and all the responsibilities which come with it. Nevertheless, one can never predict how the emotions are going to play out; especially when the surrogate has been carrying a baby for nine months. Some 'preparing for loss' work needs to be undertaken before the baby arrives, but some support and another session (or more) may be needed after the birth – even up to a year afterwards; especially when birthday blues can occur.

Not knowing a child

Some men may have walked away from a pregnancy earlier in their life; and many will feel deep regret as they have matured. The new pregnancy may bring up thoughts (and subsequent dilemmas) about trying to find the previous partner and baby he has never known.

Loss of relationships and contact

Life is rarely straightforward and fairy-tale endings do not always happen. Hypno-therapists know only too well that life can be complicated and often there are many unresolved issues concerning present and past relationships. Although mum may be happy or content in her current relationship and may be very pleased about the preg-nancy, she may have had a previous relationship which was more exciting, meaningful or rewarding than the current one. Some people settle for contentment or a 'safe' rela-tionship rather than excitement and the 'dangerous' relationship. There may be a lot of 'what-if's and regrets which arise and need to be talked about and worked through.

The following two chapters contain scripts which will help the hypnotherapist to work with some of the issues discussed above. 'The angels' archway' deals with loss and bereavement, whereas 'Letting go of baby' is for clients who are not going to keep their baby after s/he has been born.

Notes

1 Kubler-Ross, E. (1969) *On Death and Dying.* London: Routledge.
2 Parkes, C.M. and Markus, A. (1998) *Coping with Loss.* London: BMJ Books.
3 Kubler-Ross has written numerous texts but I would recommend: *On Grief and Grieving: Finding the Meaning of Grief through the 5 Stages of Loss.* London: Simon and Schuster (2014). Parkes also has written many texts but I would suggest reading his latest edition of his work with Holly Prigerson: *Bereavement: Studies of Grief in Adult Life.* London: Penguin.

42 The angels' archway

Introduction

This script should be used when the hypnotherapist knows that the client believes in some form of after-life. Some clients may follow a religion and believe in some sort of heaven, whereas others may believe there is something after life here on earth but they do not know what exactly. Some may believe in spirits and spirit guides; others may believe the soul becomes a form of energy in some way. Some clients definitely believe in angels.

The script can be used for mum, dad or birthing partner who has experienced some form of loss or bereavement. They may not have come to terms with the loss or they may still be grieving. I have found in my own practice this script works particularly well for women who have had several miscarriages. There may be a fear that they will never be able to have a baby or the terrible feeling of loss may be combined with a strong desire to speak with the babies. Very often all the lost babies come through the archway together and some very powerful work can be undertaken to help mum and her babies communicate. It should not be forgotten that a miscarriage can also affect dad, who may need support to work through the loss. Another typical experience that may be presented to the hypnotherapist is one of stillbirth or a child who has died. The script facilitates speaking to the baby or child who has been lost and so aids the grieving process.

I have found when working with women who have had several miscarriages that once this script has been used to work on the loss and bereavement, it is really helpful to do some work on strengthening the muscles surrounding the womb. This has sometimes quickly resulted in another pregnancy (which was unexpected or prior to undergoing IVF – which was then not needed) and going full-term.

The script

People who believe that there is something after this life can imagine it in different ways. Some people believe in some kind of energy, others in spirit and some people believe in angels. I know you believe there is something, so let's see where your imagination takes you.

Just close your eyes and start to relax as you know how to do so well. Take good deep breaths. Breathing in relaxes you – breathing out relaxes you even more. Breathing in relaxation – breathing out any worries or stress you have brought into the room with you today. That's right. Breathe in – and breathe out. Breathe in – and breathe out.

DOI: 10.4324/9781003173779-42

(Guidance note: when working with mum insert the following:

When you relax – your baby relaxes with you. You want to be relaxed for both you and your baby. You want to deal with things that have been bothering you – like the loss of (insert as appropriate)

Just keep relaxing – going deeper and deeper. Just imagine that you are walking along some soft green grass – there are trees on either side of you. Trees in front of you – far into the distance. You feel safe amongst the trees and with each step that you take you feel more relaxed. The leaves on the trees are rustling – you feel a gentle brush of breeze on your cheeks. So relaxing and you feel such an extraordinary sense of peace and tranquillity – all around you and inside you.

As you keep walking along the soft green grass you see an opening in the far distance. You see what looks like fluffy white clouds. You keep walking and as you get nearer and nearer the opening, you feel even more peaceful and tranquil. You also feel deep within you a sense of expectation – as though you are on your way to meet someone.

You are very near the opening now – you see lots of fluffy white clouds grouped together. Go through the opening and step onto a cloud. Lie or sit down on the cloud – whatever feels most comfortable for you. Now imagine that you are closing your eyes as you are on the cloud. I am going to start to count from *10* down to *1* – and with each number I say you will feel as though the cloud is taking you downwards.

10: Just relax and start your journey downwards
9: Going down
8: Feeling relaxed and enjoying the journey
7: Feeling very peaceful
6: Enjoying the tranquillity
5: Down and down you go
4: Going deeper and deeper
3: Letting go of any worries or stresses
2: Relaxing more and more
1: Enjoying the peace and tranquillity. When I say zero you will step off the cloud
0.

Step off the cloud and you will find yourself in a beautiful garden – this is the garden of peace and tranquillity. You may see some flowerbeds – maybe some shrubs, flowers – all neatly laid out. I wonder what else you might see – some places where you can go to sit quietly. As you are looking around you feel even more deeply this immense feeling of peace and tranquillity. Breathe in the peace and tranquillity – the depths of which you have never experienced before. Just keep breathing in deeply the peace and tranquillity.

Now suddenly in front of you, you see a mass of golden light. You feel some warmth coming from this mass of golden light – you feel energy coming from the mass of golden light. The mass of golden light does not blur your vision – you are able to look deeply into the mass of golden light. You feel energised and as you continue to look into the mass of golden light you see some movement. The more you watch the movement you can see a golden staircase more clearly – a beautiful golden staircase. Look at the bottom step – and then look up towards the top of the golden staircase. You see figures – I wonder how many you can see. You see big wings spanning out from the figures. You realise you are looking at angels.

At the top of the staircase where the angels are standing, there is an arch that goes high above the angels – from one side of the golden staircase to the other. This is the angels' archway. Keep looking at the angels. The angels are becoming clearer the more you look at them standing under the archway. You see the angels very clearly now and they have someone standing in between them – someone who is not an angel – you then realise it is *(name of baby/person who has been lost)*.

(Guidance note: if mum has had several miscarriages, stillbirths or losses, the hypnotherapist may prefer to see who appears between the angels. So, the following alternative can be used:

You see the angels very clearly now and they have people standing between them – people who are not angels – do you know who these people are)

The angels start walking down the golden staircase. *(Name)* is walking in between them. Coming down the staircase. Walk forward now and be ready to greet *(name)* at the bottom of the golden staircase. Go forward and greet *(name)*.

Now find somewhere in the garden of peace and tranquillity where you would like to spend some time with *(name)*. The angels will drift away to somewhere else in the garden – always there if you need them for anything. So now you can spend some time with *(name)* – see how s/he is – tell *(name)* whatever you need to tell him/her – ask any questions to get the answers you need.

(Guidance note: from this point on it is important that mum talks to whoever she has lost. She may be able to do this very easily or the hypnotherapist can use the prompts/questions below if needed)

What do you want to say to *(name)*?
Is there anything you want to discuss with *(name)*?
Do you have any questions for *(name)*?
Would you like to explain to *(name)* how you have been feeling?
Would you like to explain to *(name)* how losing them has affected you?
Is there anything you would like to do with *(name)*? *(e.g. if a child, play a game; if an adult, go to a place that was important/special)*
Maybe you would like to ask *(name)* how they are getting on?
What have they been doing?
How are you feeling as you are talking to *(name)*?
Can *(name)* give you any advice?
Does *(name)* want to bring anyone else through the archway and down the golden staircase to meet you?
Spend as long as you like with *(name)*. I'll be quiet until you tell me you have said and done everything you want with *(name)*. Just let me know when *(name)* is ready to go back through the archway.
As you watch *(name)* climb the golden staircase and go through the archway, feel at peace with yourself knowing that *(name)* is at peace.

(Guidance note: the hypnotherapist can ask the following question if s/he thinks further work needs to be done with someone else)

Is there anyone else you would like the angels to bring through the archway and down the golden staircase?

43 Letting go of baby

Introduction

One of the subject areas which is just not given enough attention on general hypno-therapy training or in hypnobirthing is that of loss. There can be so many types of loss and in the previous chapter the script addressed bereavement. In this chapter, I want to consider situations where mum might have to let go of her baby immediately or quite soon after the birth. Typical situations being a mum who:

- knows her baby is going to be taken into care as soon as s/he is born
- is going to have her baby adopted
- is being forced to let someone else in the family bring up her baby
- is a surrogate and who has agreed to give the baby to the intended parents.

The majority of women who choose to be a surrogate do not take on the responsibility without giving the matter an enormous amount of thought and then making detailed arrangements with the intended parents. However she approaches the surrogacy, there can be times when a surrogate has regrets or she starts to dread the thought of having to hand over the baby. The hypnotherapist may be the person the surrogate confides in and individual sessions might be booked to work on the feelings.

The same sort of feelings can arise for a mum who had decided to put her baby up for adoption. Again, this decision will not have been taken lightly in most cases, but there will be cases where mum has been forced to go down the adoption route. Mum may be forced to lie to the professionals, for example, saying she wants the adoption to take place but the reality is she does not; she has been put under pressure by the family to do so. Again, it could be the hypnotherapist who is the trusted professional and re-ceives the disclosure either before or after the birth (even months or years afterwards). In some cultures, young girls who become pregnant may be told that another member/ branch of the family will bring up the child (perhaps in another country).

A very different scenario is the mum who has been involved with Children's Social Care and knows that her baby will be taken into care immediately after the birth. She has no choice in the matter and may be experiencing a whole gamut of emotions – including anger. It needs to be said dad and other family members could be angry or upset too, and the script can be adapted for use with them.

Clients in any of the above situations need help and support and it is highly unlikely that the issues and coming to terms with letting the baby go will be resolved in one session. Intense therapy will usually be required and a qualified hypnotherapist will

DOI: 10.4324/9781003173779-43

be able to use methods and techniques they have been trained in to work on thoughts, feelings and behaviours. What I wanted to include here was a script which facilitates letting go. It is useful to record this as a track for mum (or dad/other person) so she can use it at home in between sessions.

The script

I know you are going through a difficult time at the moment and you keep thinking about the baby and how you are going to have to let him/her go after s/he is born. I want you take some time now while you are relaxed in trance to think about your thoughts and feelings. Being honest with yourself about how you feel is the first step to working on how you are going to cope with letting the baby go.

For now, just concentrate on relaxing. You know how to do this – just keep your eyes closed and let your mind drift. Let your mind relax – slow your breathing down. Breathe very slowly – in – and then out. Do that now – breathe in – and then out. As you breathe out just feel that sense of letting go. Letting go of everything that is troubling you. As you let go you feel calmer. I want you to experience and enjoy some true relaxation. You deserve this. Time for yourself. Time to think about yourself. Time to think about how you feel now – how you want to feel in the future. Time to think about what you want to do when you let go of the baby. For now, keep letting go of anything that is causing you pain or discomfort emotionally. Feel calmer and calmer. Breathe in – and breathe out – letting go – feeling calmer – more relaxed. That's really good. Keep letting go.

As you are letting go even more – you are becoming more relaxed and so much calmer. So, as you are feeling calmer, I want you to go somewhere in your mind where you feel very safe. Safe to think about things – safe to think about letting go of thoughts and feelings – and become at peace with yourself. Go to that place now.

Through life you make a lot of decisions – some which are good and some which are not so good or what you may think of as a bad decision. A bad decision is not all bad – there is always a benefit to be gained from it – you learn from it. There are times in life when decisions are made for you – decisions are taken away from you – you may not even have a say in the matter. You feel powerless – like you have no control. These situations can make you feel many different emotions – maybe sad – angry – frustrated – irritated. Or maybe you cut off your emotions and feel numb. I do not know – everyone will have their own way of dealing with things. You know how you feel and how you deal with situations and how you make decisions. Maybe you make decisions quickly – in haste. Or maybe you take your time – you think a lot – you reflect – maybe you dither or change your mind – but you get there eventually. A decision is made.

A decision has been made about what is going to happen to the baby after s/he is born. Maybe you made that decision yourself or maybe the decision was taken away from you – you feel you were forced to make that decision. Whatever has happened you know you have to let go of the baby – and you can do this. You can let go and feel that it is the right thing to do. Over the next few weeks and months, you will come to accept the decision and release any negative feelings you have about letting go of the baby.

I want you think about a time in the future when you have to let go of the baby. You know you can do this – you are going to be calm and relaxed – and strong. You have a lot of strength embedded deep down inside you – acknowledge that now. Feel that strength deep within you. You can feel and achieve anything you want. You want to be calm and relaxed when you let go of the baby. For now, think about when this is going happen – imagine the scene and let any negative feelings float in front of you. See those feelings clearly – directly in front of you – see them for what they are – unhelpful. Visualise how each of those feelings looks. Sense those feelings in front of you.

(Guidance note: the hypnotherapist can choose to do more intensive work at this point in the script, that is, talk about each negative feeling separately before getting rid of it)

Now let them go – get rid of them. Make sure they vanish completely. Let go of all those feelings. That's right – see them go now. They are gone.

You have let go of the feelings that have been unhelpful to you. You are a strong person and you have made a difficult decision *(or had to accept a decision which has been made for you)*. You have immense courage and that courage will carry you forward into the future where you can be happy and you can live your life as you wish to do.

(Guidance note: if working with a mum/parent who is having the baby taken away from them, they may resent that decision. In some cases, there may be a chance that the mum/parent has been told they may be able to get the baby back if they make changes in their life. In these cases, the hypnotherapist may wish to insert the following:

You may not be happy with the decision that has been made for you but you know what has happened in the past and the reason the decision has been made. This does not mean it has to be the end. Decisions can be changed/reversed in the future. You can choose to work on addressing certain problems (insert actual problem if known) and you can change things. You can change the way you think, feel and behave. You can be determined and motivated to show people how you can make the changes you know are required. You will not give up)

You know when you let go of the baby you are going to remain calm and relaxed but at the same time you will be acutely aware of your inner strength. Imagine that now – handing over the baby. Feel calm and relaxed – and strong. See how you look – calm and relaxed – and strong. You know you can do this. You are letting go now – you are feeling calm and relaxed – and strong. Is there anything else you want to feel? *(insert as appropriate: acceptance; at peace; resilient; proud)*. Well done – you can let go. Over the next few weeks and months see yourself letting go of the baby. See yourself letting go and as you do so, you see yourself being calm and relaxed – and very, very strong.

Part X
Ego boosting

44 The emotional flowerpot

Introduction

There are people who find it hard to talk about their emotions. This can be for all sorts of different reasons. Some may not have been allowed (an expectation of being seen and not heard) or encouraged to talk about themselves earlier in life or even in their current life; others are just not confident when talking about anything to do with themselves. Some very articulate people think it is a weakness to show any emotion, talk about feelings or vent in anyway. A victim of abuse will often feel ashamed about what has happened to them or they are scared that they will not be believed; or they may have been threatened. I have worked with women who still fear the perpetrators of their abuse even though they are dead. A person can be reluctant to speak purely because they believe they are not important (which they may have been told frequently and so believe it is true).

A person who finds it difficult to express themselves often finds it easier to talk about their emotions when in the trance state rather than in the conscious state. We know that it is healthier to talk about something rather than bottle it up, so hypnosis is an excellent way to achieve this. The script below can also enable someone to express their true feelings about a person or situation, which they would never say in the conscious state. A client will only talk about what they want and need to talk about; a hypnotherapist can never force someone to say or do something in trance. This should have been explained in detail to the client before and during the first session. However, I think when using this script, it is best practice to make this point again. A client will often feel very safe when in trance and when feeling this way is enabled to discuss their true feelings. It can give the client a wonderful sense of release and a shift occurs, so they feel different when they come back to the conscious state.

This script can be used as a one-off in a session to work on particular emotions, but it is also possible to return to the flowerpot in future sessions in order to build confidence. The client will see how the seeds have grown from week to week. It is also an effective way of assessing the client's emotional wellbeing. The script can be used for mum, dad or birthing partner, but it is presented below for mum.

The script

I want you to imagine that you are in a beautiful garden and somewhere in the garden there is a large greenhouse. So just have a wander around the garden. Enjoy looking at

DOI: 10.4324/9781003173779-44

the flowers, shrubs, whatever else might be there for you to delight in – while you look for a greenhouse. Take your time – tell me when you have found it.

The greenhouse will have lots of things growing in it – bulbs, plants, flowers and vegetables. It will also have gardening equipment and other things that are needed to help growth. It is important that seeds and plants are nurtured so that they will grow and thrive. Have a good look around and be aware of all the things that are in the greenhouse. Take your time – get to know what is in the greenhouse.

When you are ready, I want you to find an empty flowerpot. Take your time because you need to find the right flowerpot. You will know which is the right flowerpot once you see it. Tell me when you have found it. Now tell me what your flowerpot looks like.

OK – pick up the flowerpot and somewhere in the greenhouse there will be a table on which you can place it. This flowerpot is different to other flowerpots because it grows feelings. I know that you sometimes find it hard to *(insert as appropriate, e.g. talk about certain things; find the right words; express how you feel)*. I also know that you are worried that you might not love or feel anything for your baby *(or insert other worry)*. So your emotional flowerpot is going to help you with this.

Right are you ready? I want you to find some things in the greenhouse that might help you to nurture and grow things in your flowerpot. Have a good look around. I know somewhere in the greenhouse you are going to find some very powerful potting compost and a trowel. The powerful potting compost has lots of ingredients to make things grow very quickly and whatever grows in the compost will be strong and sturdy. Tell me when you have found the powerful potting compost and trowel. Have you found anything else whilst you have been looking around?

Now just stand easily by the table with the flowerpot in front of you. Look deep into the empty flowerpot. Look deep down into the very centre of it. Just relax – do not force anything – just let your thoughts drift into the flowerpot. Start thinking about how you would like to feel in the future. Maybe think about a feeling you have never had before – one you would like to feel now or in the future. Or a feeling you have experienced in the past and would like to have that feeling again and again. Just let those thoughts about feelings drift into your subconscious mind and into the flowerpot.

Tell me what feelings you are thinking about.

(Guidance note: it does not matter if mum only expresses one feeling. This is common for a mum who is very shy or finds it difficult to express her emotions initially. If mum does think about more than one feeling, the hypnotherapist should make a note of each feeling expressed. It is also good to encourage mum to talk more about the feelings and why she wants to experience them)

OK so we have: *(list/repeat the feeling(s) discussed)*.

Now would be a good time to put some powerful potting compost in the flowerpot. When you have done that have a look around the greenhouse again and find a packet of seeds. Bring the packet to the table and open it. Take one seed out of the packet now. Take the seed and plant *(insert feeling)*. Experience that feeling as you are putting it into the flowerpot. Surround it with a little more powerful potting compost. That's right.

(Guidance note: if mum has identified more than one feeling she would like to have, the hypnotherapist should then help her to plant one seed at a time – one seed for each emotion. The hypnotherapist should say each feeling out loud)

Now take another seed and plant *(insert feeling)*. Experience that feeling as you are putting it into the flowerpot. Surround it with a little more powerful potting compost.

(Guidance note: mum will keep going until all the seeds have been planted. For a mum who is worried she might not have any feeling for her baby the hypnotherapist can use the following question:
What would you like to feel for your baby?

The feeling(s) would then be planted in the same way as above)

Just make sure you have enough powerful potting compost in the flowerpot. Now have a look around for a small watering can and there should be a tap somewhere in the garden. When you have found the can, fill it up and then pour some water into the flowerpot. As you are pouring the water from the can, you are feeling a sense of newness – the beginning of something which will grow and thrive.

Now find the right place in the greenhouse to put your flowerpot. It needs to be in the right place – it needs to feel right. Find the right place now. Good. Just make sure that you know where the watering can is and also there will be a bottle of feeder – full of nutrients. Place that near the flowerpot too. Over the next few days and weeks, you are going to nurture the seeds and watch them grow. Just like you are nurturing your baby as s/he is growing inside of you.

For now though, just imagine that you are standing looking at the flowerpot. Imagine that the seeds are growing. They are just starting to pop up through the compost. They are growing up higher – looking strong and sturdy.

Tell me what *(insert feeling)* looks like. Now feel it inside of you.

Tell me what *(insert feeling)* looks like. Now feel it inside of you.

(Guidance note: the hypnotherapist will guide mum through all the feelings/seeds planted)

So, you see, you can feel emotions – you can experience different feelings and talk about them. All you have to do is imagine your flowerpot.

(Guidance note: the hypnotherapist will then get mum to anchor the flowerpot)

45 Superwoman

Introduction

A common theme through this book is how to address a lack of confidence. A deficit of confidence can stem from many things but often it is the fear of the unknown. Attention has also been given to the fact that a mum may be told all sorts of old wives' tales or horror stories about bad experiences in childbirth. As an alternative to all the negative stories, it is important to talk about good experiences and also to remember people who are positive or have been influential in the past. The objective of the superwoman script is to help mum build confidence in herself by remembering good role models she has had in her life. However, a word of caution is needed because some mums may not have had any good influences in their life (especially if they have a history of abuse or have been in the care system). Therefore, the hypnotherapist may need to encourage mum to think about people she admires from afar rather than people she knows or has had direct contact with in her own life. The script helps mum to develop skills and ideally should be returned to in future sessions.

Within the script I have included a lot of questions and prompts. When planning the session with mum, it is important that the hypnotherapist leaves plenty of time for responses and to undertake in-depth work.

The script

I wonder how you see yourself? Just picture an image of you now. What do you see? When you look at that image – what do you feel? Is that image the real you? Do you sometimes put on a front? Are you good at acting and performing for others? Do you hide your true feelings from other people? You know that you can be any way you want to be. You understand and believe in the power of your subconscious mind. You have so much strength deep inside, you can conquer anything that is holding you back.

Just keep focussing on that image of you. In a moment I want you to change that image. I want you to change that image of you – you are still you – but on the count of *3* you are going to become you the superwoman. *1, 2,* and *3* – see you the superwoman.

Look at you the superwoman closely. We all have different images of what it is like to be superwoman. Some people immediately think about superwoman in the comics – wearing her blue and red outfit with a huge letter 'S' on her front. But superwomen come in all different shapes and sizes. Look at how you the superwoman looks. Tell me what you see.

DOI: 10.4324/9781003173779-45

As you are looking at you the superwoman let your mind drift back to women you have met in your life – women you have admired – women you have come to respect. Also think about superwomen who have influenced you from afar *(special emphasis is needed here if it is known mum has not had many positive role models/influences in her life)*. Go right back to childhood – think about who the superwomen were at that time in your life. Who did you admire? Who did you respect? Now think about adolescence. Who were the superwomen at that time in your life? Who did you admire? Who did you respect? Now into adulthood – who have been the superwomen in your life? Who have you admired? Who have you respected? Who are the superwomen in your life now? Who do you admire? Who do you respect?

Think about all these wonderful women. Bring all these superwomen together in a group – see them sitting in a group in front of you. How many women are there? Look at each one in turn – consider what it is about each woman that you admire and respect. Think about the strengths and qualities each woman possesses. I am going to be quiet for a little while now – so you can think about each individual superwoman – her strengths and her qualities. Imagine that you have a notebook and pen in your hands. As you are looking and thinking about each individual superwoman make a list in your notebook of all her strengths and qualities you admire and respect. Tell me when you have finished your list – after considering each superwoman in the group.

(Guidance note: the hypnotherapist should remember to leave a good length of time for this activity in the first session but can come back at the next session to check whether mum has remembered any other superwomen)

Now look at the list and tell me about the strengths and qualities of your superwomen.

You already have a lot of inner strength yourself and in the next few months until your baby is born you will be facing new situations and you will experience new thoughts and feelings. You may question things and sometimes you may worry about things – that is only natural. When you are uncertain or worried about something, you need to feel your inner strength and believe in yourself. You know you can be you the superwoman who is strong and confident.

Look again at the list you have written about your superwomen's strengths and qualities. Tell me which ones you think you have got already. Then think about which ones you need to develop for the future – during your pregnancy and for birthing. Make a new list in the notebook. When you are ready tell me which strengths and qualities you want you the superwoman to have.

Imagine now, superwoman from the comics. She is wearing her blue top with the big red letter 'S' on it, skirt and tights. This superwoman is known for her super powers – immense unlimited strength – being able to fly – speed – an enhanced sense of sight. Superwoman's strength comes from deep within her but she also has incredible strength in her legs and arms – this helps her fly at great speed.

Stay with the comic superwoman and just imagine her ready to go into action. See how she looks – confident, determined and ready. She is thinking about her mission – look at her face – see the deep concentration mixed with confidence – knowing that she is going to achieve her mission. She bends her knees – ready for action – and then up she goes – jumping in the air – going so high – as high as she needs to be. She is up in the air now – see how fast she flies – going exactly where she needs to go.

Now look at you the superwoman.

(Guidance note: the hypnotherapist should ask the following three questions initially and then, if mum says that superwoman does need to increase her strengths or add qualities, mum should be encouraged to bring in changes to the image and anchor the strength/quality)

When dressed as you the superwoman, what are you wearing?
How are you the superwoman looking?
Tell me what qualities you like most about you the superwoman.

Look again now at the second list you made – the strengths and qualities you want to develop. Imagine you have developed these strengths and qualities. Look at you the superwoman again.
What has changed about you the superwoman?
What are you the superwoman wearing?
How are you the superwoman looking?

Look a little closer and you will see that superwoman is wearing a belt around her waist. This belt is her toolkit and it has the power to expand. In the toolkit there are all sorts of equipment and other things – including knowledge, experience, skills – all of which can be expanded in the toolkit, but new knowledge, experiences and skills can be added at any time.
Would you like to add anything to your superwoman's toolkit? You can add anything at all. If, so add them now.

(Guidance note: the hypnotherapist should work in-depth with mum as she adds to her toolkit)

Look at you the superwoman – see how strong you are – see how well prepared you are – ready to face any new situation. Now feel as you the superwoman – feel the strength and confidence – ready to face anything new – you are prepared. You have the knowledge, experience and skills in your toolkit. Your toolkit can help you to achieve anything you want to do. To get something you need out of the toolkit, all you have to do is think about what you need and tap the toolkit twice. Do that now.

(Guidance note: at this point the hypnotherapist can continue to address certain situations which need to be worked on or, in a future session, superwoman can be returned to work on particular issues/situations. Superwoman can be useful when using her super powers for:

Distraction: flying anywhere
Bonding: flying with baby
Making time go faster: using superwoman's power of speed
Stopping pain: strength to move walls/barriers to pain)

46 The rocky mountain

Introduction

This script is about being on the right path and being able to deal with any obstacles that try to take mum off track. It is about the determination to carry on and succeed. It embeds the idea that mum will know instinctively the right way to go and the right thing to do. What is also a very important message is that it is perfectly fine to change direction at any time. This script works really well with a group, but more in-depth work can be achieved when used in individual sessions. At the end of the script mum can be left to do some bonding with baby.

The script

Sometimes in life it can feel that what you really want or want to be is impossible to achieve. It can feel like the world is working against you – every obstacle possible is put in your way. Even though you keep on trying, you start to lose your energy and feel getting what you want is just downright impossible. So, you might start to feel lethargic, unmotivated and question yourself – 'Why bother?' Feelings like this can come and go. It is so important to believe in yourself and know that you can achieve anything if you really want to do so.

I would like you to imagine that you are standing at the bottom of a huge rocky mountain. It is the highest rocky mountain you have ever seen. It is a very beautiful mountain because there are so many interesting shapes, things to see as you look at the rocks that are on the mountain. The rocky mountain is so very high, it looks like it is reaching into the sky. Even though it is very high, you can still see the very top of the rocky mountain. Look at the top of the rocky mountain now and see your baby – right at the very top. Lying comfortably waiting for you. Your baby is smiling and laughing and waiting for you.

Now I know you sometimes feel very tired and everything is such an effort. Sometimes you may doubt yourself – you may feel you cannot get through this pregnancy or be a good mum *(or insert any particular doubts/issues mum has talked about)*. Whenever you doubt yourself in the future, I want you to imagine the rocky mountain. Imagine that you are standing at the bottom of the rocky mountain just like you are doing now.

Just stay very still at the bottom of the rocky mountain. Take some deep, slow breaths – breathe in – *1, 2,* and *3.* Good – now breathe out – *3, 2,* and *1.* Keep breathing at a nice slow pace. Breathing in and out will relax you and help you face any rock that might come at you. On this mountain some of the rocks are loose and they can have

DOI: 10.4324/9781003173779-46

a tendency to fall off the mountain and down the side. It may feel like the rocks are trying to stop you getting to the top. The rocks may try to divert you from the route you have chosen to take, but you know that you can get to the top of the rocky mountain – you can reach the very top and meet your baby.

You are well-equipped for this climb to the top, so nothing is going to stop you. Just look at what you are wearing. You have a helmet to protect your head if any rocks start coming down from above. This is a very special helmet because it also protects you from any negative comments or old wives' tales that you may hear. It also keeps in your own positive thoughts, your mantras and affirmations. So, you can always imagine you are wearing this helmet no matter where you are. You can see and feel it around your head, but it is invisible to everyone else.

You are wearing a harness around your waist, where your climbing rope is threaded through the loops. You also have a safety chain. Your climbing rope and safety chain are there to keep you safe – you will not fall. Now look at your climbing boots – they are designed just for climbing – they grip really hard. You will not slip on the rocks. You have a chalk bag and chalk tied to your harness, so if your hands become hot and sweaty, you can use the chalk to make them dry – get a better hold of things.

Right, you are ready to go. You are going to climb the rocky mountain to the very top, where your baby is waiting for you. Have a quick look up there – see how your baby is smiling and laughing – waiting for you. On the count of *3* start climbing – *1, 2, and 3*. Start climbing.

Start slowly at first – feeling your way. It is wise to take your time and feel your way when you are doing something you have not done before. So, feel your way with your hands and feet. You will know instinctively the best route for you to reach the very top of the rocky mountain to reach your baby. When you want to achieve something, there is nothing wrong with taking time to feel your way – ask questions, do the research, stop and reflect on what you are told and what you learn. There is never any need to make a hasty decision – you need to achieve your goals in a timescale that suits you – not others. So, take your time climbing the rocky mountain. Stop and start if you need to – think about the best route to take.

Let your hands and feet explore the rocks as you climb higher and higher. You know instinctively the best route up to the top of the rocky mountain. Sometimes it may be necessary to change direction. Things can happen which make another route the better way. With each step you take up the mountain, you feel more confident – knowing which is the best route for you to reach your baby. Keep climbing – change the route if you need to do so – keep climbing to reach your baby at the very top of the mountain.

Enjoy the climb. Keep focussed on reaching the very top. I wonder what emotions you are feeling as you continue climbing to reach your baby at the very top – excitement – exhilaration – so proud of yourself.

You can take a rest whenever you want to – you do not have to do the climb without taking a break – take some time to think about the route you are climbing. You might want to stop and take a look out across the world. You are bringing new life into the world – such a tremendous and worthwhile thing to do. So just stop now and look out. Feel good about the world – feel good about your life – feel good about you and your baby. If anything comes into your mind that is not helpful to you – a particular thought – a belief – a feeling – any self-doubt about your capabilities *(insert anything else which might be appropriate for mum)* – just throw whatever it is off the side of the rocky mountain – never to be seen again.

Good – you are ready to continue your climb. Keep climbing – feeling good – feeling confident that you can reach the very top of the rocky mountain. That's right. Let your hands and feet feel the right way to get to the top.

Suddenly some dust falls on your face and into your eyes. You wipe it away – nothing is going to distract you from your route. Keep climbing upwards. Then you hear a rumbling sound; you hear it again. You realise it is the sound of rocks falling down from higher up the rocky mountain. The rocks are like people in life who try to derail you – who may say unhelpful things to you – they do not encourage you – they do not support you in the ways you need. You are prepared for the falling rocks – you know what to do. You can see the rocks coming – so you swing out of the way quickly to avoid them – holding tightly onto your climbing rope – not letting go – holding on tightly. Your climbing boots are gripping the side of the rocky mountain. Gripping hard – you are not going to fall. The rocks keep coming but you are prepared; you can deal with any obstacle that comes your way. You stay calm and strong – nothing will deter you.

The falling rocks seem to get fewer now. Fewer and fewer. You use your hands to push the smaller rocks out of your way. You are steadfast – you stay just where you are until the rocks have stopped falling.

OK – now continue the rest of your climb. Enjoy it – you have nothing to fear. You can deal with anything that comes at you. You know exactly which way you are going. You are confident in the route you are taking. Getting to the top of the rocky mountain on a route that is right for you. Feeling safe because you know you have your helmet, harness, climbing rope, safety chain, chalk bag and climbing boots.

You are nearly there now – looking forward to reaching the top of the mountain where your baby is waiting for you. Keep climbing – only a short way to go now. And you are there – hoist yourself on to the top of the mountain. Go and pick up your baby – give him/her a cuddle. Sit down with your baby on top of the mountain. Look down the side of the rocky mountain – see how far you have climbed – congratulate yourself. The falling rocks did not deter you from reaching the top of the rocky mountain. Be proud of yourself – what you have achieved.

Look out from the rocky mountain – across to the world. Show your baby the world. Talk to your baby about your hopes and aspirations for the future. Spend some relaxing time now talking to your baby.

47 You can so do this

Introduction

The simple objective of the following script is to work on self-belief by ego boosting. In earlier chapters, mention has been made of the fact that some mums may not welcome the pregnancy. In many situations, this is because mum does not believe she is capable of being a good mum or thinks she will not be able to cope; her self-esteem might be low and she may be lacking in confidence. This script can be used in its own right or towards the end of an individual session when other work has been undertaken. It is a very powerful script when used with a group – especially younger girls.

The script

I know that you doubt yourself a lot. You don't think you are capable of achieving much. Maybe you have been told you are – useless – stupid – daft *(or if known, insert any other negative word(s) that has/have been used)* and you have come to believe it. Have you ever thought about how many times in a day or a week you say, 'I can't'? Or how many times you say something negative about yourself: 'I'm going to fail' *(or insert a particular phrase if known).* How many times in a day or a week do you put yourself down? Now is the time to stop the negative thoughts and language – and to start believing in yourself. You have started this already – you have taken the step to come here – that took a lot of courage. That was a big step and shows you want to make changes in your life. You can so do this.

So, while you are resting comfortably there, I want you to think about things you want to achieve in the future for yourself and for your baby. Think about what is really important to you. Think about what is holding you back. What is it that is making you doubt yourself? You know that if you really want to achieve something – you will achieve it – if you are really determined to do so. You need to believe in yourself and I want you to start saying to yourself more and more, 'I can so do this'. This is going to be your new mantra: 'I can so do this'.

You have learnt lots of things yourself from the moment you were born. Well actually, even before you came into the world you knew what to do – you knew how to live in the womb and how to be born. You knew the journey you had to take to come into the world. Through your childhood you learnt things – at home – at school – maybe from other people in different places. You started to achieve things from a very early age. You learnt in childhood and you continued to learn as a young person and will continue to learn all through your adulthood. You never ever stop learning. You are

DOI: 10.4324/9781003173779-47

coming to these sessions to learn how to use hypnosis to help with your pregnancy and birthing. You can so do this – enjoy your pregnancy and give birth to your baby easily.

(Guidance note: if working in an individual session the hypnotherapist can insert other objectives mum might be working on)

You are a very unique individual. You do not have to be like other people and do things as they do. You can choose to do things in your own way – the way that is best for you. You just need to believe in yourself – believe you can do whatever you want to do. You can so do this.

Imagine that you are in a sports stadium. You are standing on a running track. There are hurdles to be jumped over all around the track. You are dressed for running. Look down at your front – instead of seeing a number like most athletes have on their vest you see your mantra written, 'I can so do this'. Now crouch down on the track and get ready for your run around the track – you are going to jump very high over all those hurdles with ease. Think about what you want to achieve in the future – for you and for your baby. Think about what has been stopping you in the past – the reasons that have caused you not to believe in yourself. See any words, phrases or people that have hindered you in the past or in the present, painted on the hurdles in front of you. See them clearly painted on the hurdles. You are going to run around the track and jump very high over each hurdle. So, look at each hurdle and see what has been holding you back and know for sure that you can jump over any hurdle in front you. You can jump as high as you like. You can so do this.

On your starter's orders – ready – steady – go. Start running and jump high over each hurdle. Jump as high as you need to – you can so do this. Keep running. Keep jumping as high as you can – as high as you need to. You can so do this. Believe in yourself as you are running round the track. You know you can jump high over each hurdle. You can achieve anything you really want to do. Nothing and no-one is going to hold you back. Round you go. You can so do this. You see the finish line and run over it. You have so done it.

Take some deep breaths. You have used a lot of energy running around the track and jumping high over all the hurdles. Now you are going to go around the track again. You are suddenly aware the stadium has filled up now with spectators. Look down at your front and see your mantra, 'I can so do this'. On your starter's orders – ready – steady – go. Start running and prepare to jump high over each hurdle. Jump as high as you need to – you can so do this. As you face the first hurdle, you take a quick look at the spectators in the stadium – remarkably they all look like you. Over the hurdle you go. Keep going towards the next hurdle. You look at the spectators again – they all look like you. You hear them shouting, 'You can so do this'. Over the hurdle you go – so high and so easily. Keep going round the track – jumping high over the hurdles. Hear the spectators shouting loud and clear, 'You can so do this'. The spectators believe in you – you believe in yourself. You can achieve anything you want. You can so do this.

(Guidance note: the hypnotherapist can choose to embed specific goals at this point)

You are going to go through the rest of your pregnancy with confidence, because you believe in yourself. You will be able to birth your baby easily because you believe in yourself. You will be a good parent because you believe in yourself. You can so do this.

48 The ballerina

Introduction

The ballerina is a metaphor which can be used to build mum's confidence. It works well with mums who may have experienced abuse, bullying or received little attention or support from their family. Consequently, they may be lacking in confidence and their self-esteem may be extremely low, so that they are questioning their abilities to get through the pregnancy and birthing. This metaphor also includes some imagery regarding stretching and staying focussed which can aid the birthing process. The ultimate objective of this script is ego-boosting.

The script

Today I want you to think about some of the conversations we have had previously about being relaxed, in control of your mind and body, how they are connected and also how the uterus muscles work in pregnancy and during birthing. You know it is important to keep fit both in your mind and body, and when in trance to practise stretching both your mind and body.

So, I want to tell you about a young girl who became a ballerina. I think you might find it helpful to visualise the ballerina and her graceful movements but first let me tell you about the young girl, who I shall call the ballerina. The ballerina had not had a happy childhood at all. She lived with her parents and three brothers. Her parents were always arguing and fighting, and her three brothers always sided with their dad rather their mum. The ballerina did not like all the shouting and noise, and she felt very alone when her mum died when she was just a young girl. Although her brothers were very cruel to her, the ballerina always felt it was her responsibility to look after them – even though she was the youngest.

The ballerina did love to dance and she used to lose herself in her dance to escape the horrible things she saw and heard happening in her house. When she danced, she went into a trance. Her dad and her brothers made fun of her when she used to dance around the house but it was her way of escaping. The ballerina went to a local dance school and the teacher there thought she had great talent and potential. The ballerina did not feel confident and thought the dance teacher was just being kind when she said she was born to be a ballerina and she could go far. Her dad and brothers told the ballerina she would never amount to anything. The dance teacher was proven to be right – the ballerina did have talent and when she was older, she auditioned and got into a national ballet company.

DOI: 10.4324/9781003173779-48

So now imagine you are going to the theatre to see the ballerina. You are going to see just how smoothly and elegantly she dances. You are entering the theatre now. Passing the ticket office, the bar, the programme sellers and lots of people who are milling around. You have your ticket ready in your hand. I wonder if you are going to sit in the stalls, the circle or the upper circle. You know where you are going – which direction to go in to find your seat. Make your way there now and when you have found the right entrance door, hand your ticket to the person standing there. Now go and find your seat which is going to have such a good view of the stage.

The ballerina is going to perform a solo dance, which is so much harder to do than dancing with others because all the attention will be on her. Only her. She feels a great sense of responsibility that she must perform well for the audience. She must not let them down.

Make yourself comfortable in your seat. You hear people chattering away. They are excited and anticipating the performance. Have a look around and see who is sitting next to you. I wonder if anyone is sitting in any of the boxes on the sides of the stage. Look at all the lights high up – scattered around the theatre. Suddenly the lights dim and people stop talking. There is a gentle hush. Then it is completely dark. You hear the swoosh of the stage curtains draw back. A spotlight comes on – you see the centre of the stage.

The ballerina glides onto the stage. The audience applauds. Look at her beautiful tutu. What colour is it? What colour are her ballet shoes? Is she wearing anything in her hair? She takes her place centre stage – ready to start. Her head is held high. She is full of confidence. The theatre is now completely silent. Then the music starts.

Just watch the ballerina dance. All her movements are so smooth; she is so graceful – her limbs are so fluid. Now watch her carefully – see how she makes everything she does look so easy. It is as though it does not take any effort at all. Look how all her movements follow each other – how everything flows – no hesitation. This is because the ballerina knows exactly what to do. She knows what order the movements come in. She has practised for hours and hours and hours – every day – every week – every month – for years and years. Practise. Practise. Practise. So now everything happens naturally – it all flows – there is no hesitation at all.

Watch how the ballerina stretches all her muscles throughout her body. She does an arabesque. She is standing on one leg. The other leg is stretched out behind her. One arm is stretched up in the air. The other arm is stretched out behind her. Now she is opening her arms – taking them above her head – stretching them – so beautifully and easily. All the muscles are stretching naturally.

In other movements, she stretches the smaller parts of her body – she points her fingers – she points her toes. Little parts of her are so strong because she has trained them through practice to be so. Her delicate little toes are strong – she can stand on them; she can walk on them – her ballet shoes have metal built in the front of them. Her toes are strong – she has made them strong through practice. When she first used point shoes her feet and toes bled and bled; they do not do that anymore. Her toes have become strong.

Every part of the ballerina is strong – her body and her mind. She was determined to achieve what she wanted – she wanted to dance – she wanted to become a ballerina. She never gave up even though so many obstacles were put in her way and she had no support from her dad or brothers. She was determined to succeed through practice, practice and practice. Through her determination, she became stronger physically and emotionally and she did succeed – she became a ballerina.

Now the ballerina is running gracefully across the stage. She turns around, runs a little way and then takes a massive leap and soars through the air. She runs again takes another leap and goes even higher. She can go as high as she likes – soaring through the air. Her strong legs push her high up into the air. She can go as high as she wants – she knows she can achieve anything she wants to do. The ballerina is confident in her ability and skills – because she has practised.

Now she is nearing the end. She does a series of pirouettes – spinning round on one leg while her other leg is off the ground and her toes are pointing towards her knee. Round and round and round she goes, on one leg. Her mind is focussed – her eyes are focussed – she looks for one spot as she spins round and round and round. She stays focussed. She knows she can make this ending spectacular. Her eyes have found something to focus on and look for each time she spins round – she spots it each time she goes around. Round and round and round. She is going faster and faster each time she goes around. Then suddenly she stops – precisely in one position. It's all over.

The audience goes wild with excitement. The ballerina smiles, walks forward and curtsies. She is happy. She has made the audience happy, which was her goal. The ballerina never used to believe in herself because her dad and brothers had told her she would never amount to anything. She wanted to dance and become a ballerina. Through determination and practising every day she made both her mind and body strong and she came to believe in herself.

The ballerina doubted herself when she was young. She did not believe in herself at all, because her dad and brothers had told her she would not amount to anything. She proved them wrong. She was determined to succeed. I know you have had some doubts about yourself *(insert as appropriate)* but think about the ballerina now and in the future. Look how she practised – how she became strong in both her mind and body. She knew what she had to do – she prepared herself – she came to believe in herself. Even her body became very strong, her body was also very pliable and flexible – it could adapt. It could bend and stretch – move in all directions – at different speeds. She could travel in different ways – walk gracefully, run, skip, jump, leap. Your body can do the same. You can be pliable and flexible during your pregnancy and when the baby starts his/her journey into the world. You know what is going to happen – you are preparing now – you are practising – you will stay focussed. When your baby starts its journey into the world you are going to give a magnificent performance – the performance of your lifetime.

(Guidance note: the hypnotherapist should then embed some direct suggestions)

49 Sadie

Introduction

I wrote the Sadie script as a metaphor because through my working life I have met a lot of Sadies and in my role as a hypnotherapist I have worked with clients to address similar issues the metaphorical Sadie had. The script finds a place in this book because, as I stated earlier, a pregnant young girl or woman may have issues in their life which, if worked on, will help her pregnancy and future life with the baby.

This script works particularly well with very young mums (16 years and under) and anyone who has experienced abuse. It is a script that can be used in a group when working with young girls that have similar histories or experiences. It is important when running such groups that the sessions are planned so there is time for group discussion in the conscious state after the work has been done in the trance state. The discussion usually facilitates the knowledge that they are not alone in their experiences. Members of a group can grow close together and form a support system for the future.

The script

I want to tell you about Sadie because I think you might find her story interesting. I want you to imagine Sadie, who was 16 years old when she found out she was pregnant. She was a very young 16-year-old and she was very scared, but also very pleased, when she realised that she was pregnant. You see Sadie did not believe that anyone really loved her and she thought that if she had a baby, she would be able to make it love her, because she would be a good mum. When she was pregnant, she used to say: 'I'll just do the exact opposite to what my mum did. Then I'll be a good mum. I can be different'.

Sadie was living with her grandad when she found out she was pregnant. Sadie had lived with her mum when she was younger, but her mum did not look after her very well. Sadie would tell people: 'My mum never wanted me'. Sadie's mum had been in a violent relationship with Sadie's dad and would never talk about him. All her grandad would say was: 'You're better off not knowing. He wasn't a good person'. Sadie thought she could remember bits about her dad – she used to get images in her head and remember certain things – but none of it really made any sense to her.

Sadie's mum had lots of problems herself. She did not eat much but drank a lot of alcohol, which resulted in her owing money to a lot of people, including loan sharks. She used to go on drinking binges and leave Sadie on her own. Sadie was neglected a lot, which is how her grandad came to take her in eventually. Grandad had not had

DOI: 10.4324/9781003173779-49

contact with Sadie or her mum for many years; he had had no idea what had been happening to Sadie. When he found out, he felt very guilty, because he had eventually broken off contact with his daughter after years of trying to help her so many times.

When Sadie came to live with her grandad life was better in many ways, but Sadie faced new problems. Like many children who have gone for long periods of time without food, Sadie would overeat – even though she knew her grandad would never starve her. As she ate more and more, she put on a lot of weight, so a lot of the children at school made fun of her and some bullied her. Image seemed to be very important to a lot of the children at school and who lived in the local area. Sadie did not have any real friends at school and she felt very lonely.

Sadie believed she was ugly. This was a word she heard in her head; it was like a little voice telling her she was ugly and she heard the word so often she came to believe it. It did not help that Sadie suffered with eczema, so her skin was often red, sore and very itchy. She got into the habit of scratching her skin which made it much worse.

Sadie loved her grandad, who definitely loved her, but Sadie did not believe this – she did not believe she was loveable. She believed her dad had left because she was not loveable. She felt that her grandad had only taken her in because he had to, otherwise social services would have taken her into care. No matter how much her grandad tried to reassure her that was not the case and that she was loved and wanted, Sadie did not believe it. She did not believe that anyone could want her when she was so ugly.

Sadie desperately wanted to be loved. She wanted to be part of a proper family – in her head that meant having a mum, dad, brothers and sisters. She did not consider her and her grandad to be a proper family.

Sadie did not go out much because she did not have any friends. She spent most of her time in her bedroom and using the internet. She met Aron online through Facebook. They chatted for weeks before actually meeting face-to-face. Sadie met Aron twice and got pregnant. She had no idea where he lived.

Sadie was scared to tell her grandad she was pregnant, so she kept the pregnancy hidden for a long time. That was easy to do because Sadie was over-weight and she always wore baggy clothes. Although she was scared about the future, in her heart Sadie was excited about having a baby. She thought of the baby as hers and no-one else's. She started to imagine all the things she wanted to do for and with her baby. She kept thinking back to her life as a little girl and what her mum had not done for her, so she started saying to herself: 'I can be different'. She said it to herself silently in her head, but also out loud when she was alone.

Although Sadie hated being at school, she did like some of the support staff and it was one member of staff she told she was pregnant. In that school, different groups were run by counsellors and therapists. Sadie started seeing a hypnotherapist to work on her lack of confidence and low self-esteem. When in trance she could talk about things more easily and she regressed back to the awful things that had happened to her and worked through her feelings about that and how her mum had treated her. Gradually, she began to realise that none of this had been her fault. The hypnotherapist worked with Sadie to build her confidence, plan for the future and also taught her techniques to use for birthing.

Sadie felt the baby gave her a purpose and something to live for. She said she had always felt 'ugly and useless' before being pregnant. Sadie had struggled at school – she was not an academic, but she had other talents. She had always been good at making things – she was resourceful. This had come out of having to find things and make do when her mum neglected her. Sadie started making things for the baby – she knitted and sewed, but she was also good at making and restoring furniture. She was really well prepared for when she had her baby girl. After the baby was born, Sadie started doing more craftwork and eventually developed a small business which she ran from home. She still regularly said to herself: 'I can be different'.

A lot can be learnt from Sadie's story. It is important how you see yourself – not how others see you – and to believe in yourself. You can learn from what has happened in the past and make changes for the future – you just have to believe in yourself. Having a purpose or goal can help. Everyone is good at something. Everyone is talented in some way. Like Sadie, you can be different too.

50 Well done you

Introduction

This script is to be used for mum in the last class of any group or the last individual session. The main objective is to commend and congratulate mum on what she has achieved, but also to focus on ego boosting. It is a really good script to give to mum as a track or on a CD so that she can listen to it when the sessions have finished.

The script

First of all, I want to congratulate you on how well you have done in preparing for your baby's birth. It took some courage to come to the first class/session – so well done for taking that step. You should be very proud of yourself – you have achieved so much in the past few weeks – from when you first started the classes/sessions until now – and in between you have been practising so regularly. It is always a good thing to reflect on things – to acknowledge the positives and the benefits. There is no better time to do this than when you are in the trance state. So, let's do that now.

Just relax and start letting go. Letting go of anything that is circling around your mind – anything that you have been thinking about today that is not connected to you or the baby – just let everything drift away. Your normal day-to-day life – let it go. Now is the time to think about how well you have done and what you have achieved.

Every person doubts themselves at some point in their life – some do this more frequently than others. Some women will doubt that they can get through a pregnancy; others may not believe they will be a good mum and other doubts may have flashed through your mind previously *(if appropriate insert any particular doubts mum had and which have successfully been worked on – then commend her)*. Self-doubt is not a good thing and after attending these classes/sessions you do not doubt yourself at all. You know you are going through your pregnancy with a positive attitude – enjoying the pregnancy and looking forward to the birth of your baby. The word 'doubt' no longer has a place in your vocabulary or in your mind. Well done you.

You have learnt about hypnosis and how to use self-hypnosis. Just let your mind drift back to some of the things you have done in the classes/sessions or at home. Remember the good thoughts you have had and the good feelings you have experienced. Self-hypnosis has become part of your life because you have practised – practised – and practised. It will remain part of your life to promote your wellbeing – keeping you well physically – mentally – and emotionally. When the baby arrives, you will be busy and at times your body will become tired. You know that it will be beneficial to

DOI: 10.4324/9781003173779-50

take some time out and go off in your mind – somewhere where you can relax but also somewhere to re-energise. It will be important to take time out for you. You have so many strategies now to help you physically – mentally – and emotionally. You know how to use self-hypnosis to its full benefit. Using it will benefit both you and your baby. Well done you.

You have increased your confidence over the past few weeks. You know you can do anything you really want to do. Remember the mantra: imagine – believe – achieve. You have done a lot of imagining over the past few weeks – imagining times in your pregnancy – situations you might have to face – hopes and aspirations – birthing. You have learnt a great deal and practised regularly – so much so you now firmly believe that giving birth is a very natural thing – something to look forward to – and you are going to achieve it so easily. You know you can do it. You are totally confident about this and with all the positivity and strength that is embedded deep within your body and mind you are going to achieve everything you want – the birth that you want – your baby will arrive safely into this world. Well done you.

Just feel that confidence now. Enjoy it. Know it is always deep within you – it will never leave you. So, I want to congratulate you once again for everything you have achieved and everything you will achieve in the future. I want you to congratulate yourself too – do that now – be proud of yourself. Well done you.

Index

Note: Page number followed by "n" refer to end notes.

abortion 19, 201
abuse 5, 8; categories 8, 10n10; discriminatory 10n11; domestic 6; emotional 10n10; experience of 15, 224, 227; financial/material 10n11; forms of 10n11; historical 8; history of 7, 184, 201, 216; organisational 10n11; physical 10n10, 10n11; psychological 10n11; support groups 27; survivors 18, 100, 132, 184, 197; victims of 8, 18, 20, 107, 185, 191, 193, 197, 213; see also adult abuse; child abuse; sexual abuse
abused persons, fears 8–9
abusers 8, 168, 184, 213
abusive: experience 15, 224, 227; situation 8, 9
adoption 19, 91, 201, 203, 208; of baby, feelings 208, 209
adult abuse 8, 39; survivors 18
adulthood 10, 18, 182, 186, 191; learning 222; superwomen 217
Adult Social Care 9
adults 3, 84; avoiding 66; Care and Support Statutory Guidance 11n15; consent from 22; hypnotherapy 39; with learning disabilities 40; loss 202; safeguarding 9, 11n14; self-hypnosis 122; special place 207; working with 22, 39
advertising 28, 34
affirmations 109, 166–7, 187, 220
after-life belief: script 205–7; see also angels
anchor 92, 215, 218
angels: belief in 205; looking at 206
angel's archway 207; and loss 19, 204
anniversary blues 202
anxiety 5, 92, 202; groups 27; social 37
assertiveness 18, 185; technique 168
assessment 6, 21–3, 127; aim 22; charges 39; dad's 39; and fear of blood 39; for fears 82; importance of 15; individual sessions 21–3, 38; initial 30, 35, 38, 39, 58; miscarriage disclosure 202; of mum's interests 76; of mum's past 132; phobias 38; pre-birth 9,

203; questionnaire 21, 24–5; screening 35; subjects covered in 38; time taken for 38; for trance 50; see also evaluation; risk assessment

baby: adoption, feelings 208, 209; bonding with 16, 86; feelings for 7; script 114
baby communication, scripts 162–7
baby talk, script 109–10
bathroom, script 100–3
behaviour(s) 133, 209: affects on 102, 177; change 49; problems 6, 22; and thoughts 102; triggers 35; types 6
belief(s) 9: affirmation 18, 165–6; embedded 127, 151; focus on 166; negative 184; and the subconscious mind 166; see also self-belief
benefits: for baby's dad 93; concept 92; from bad decision 209; from trance state 230; future 93, 94, 131; hazards 40; of hypnosis 29, 37, 194; people on 127; therapy, in hypnosis 92; of trained hypnotherapist 34
benefits approach: methodology i, 12; script for dad 16; theory 94n1
bereavement 205, 208; see also death; loss; loss and bereavement
birthing: experience 95, 96; future 177; hospital 145; and hypnotherapy 5; metaphor 224; methodologies i; positions for 135; preparation 14–15, 29, 38, 146, 148, 156; stretching for 17
birthing at home 18, 136; script 151, 153, 154
birthing journey 14, 16, 17, 95, 103, 133–4; script 145, 148, 150, 152, 155
birthing partner 4, 7, 13, 15, 18; breathing development 16
birthing plan 17, 132–3; conscious state 132; questionnaire 135; script 133–4
birthing pool 16, 82; script 83
birthing room 153, 171; importance 145; script 18, 70–1, 133, 136, 145–7, 148

blood pressure: high and calmness 17; script 111–14
body image, script 191
body language 168, 172
body scanner: and confidence-building 107; scripts 17, 107–10
body temperature 16, 82
bonding: with baby 16, 86; on the beach 18, 161, 162; importance of 159; in message room 18; script 17, 111, 159–60, 219–21
breathing, individual sessions 58
breathing development, birthing partner 16
breathing exercises 57–8; calmness 72–4; colour breathing 59–61; counting 58–9; hypnobirthing 58; number breathing 59; ratio breathing 59; techniques 58–61; *see also* down breathing; up breathing; up and down breathing
bullying 5, 224, 228; victims 184

caesarean section 19, 134, 135, 171, 193
calmness 61; breathing exercises 72; and high blood pressure 17; and relaxation 61; script 78, 111–14; tunnel of 17, 111–14; wave of 121
Care Act (2014) 10n11, 11n14
categories, of abuse 8, 10n10
child 3; best interests of 22; life stages 86; loss of 91, 202; as mum 13; sharing information about 26; stillbirth 205; taken into care 203; told untruths 185; unknown to father 204
child abuse 8, 26, 39; categories 10n10; survivors 18
children, Safeguarding Partnership 9
Children Act (1989) 10n10, 11n14, 22, 26
Children Act (2004) 11n14, 26
cinema trip 17, 144, 145, 147, 150, 154; script 136–7, 138
concerns 21, 39, 95, 112; *see also* worries
confidence, lack of 5, 7, 15, 18, 39, 91, 184, 203, 216, 228
confidence-building 29, 77, 151, 168, 184, 213, 216; ballerina metaphor 224–5; and body scanner 107; hypnotherapy 184; scripts 19, 20, 107, 184–7, 216–18, 222; *see also* ego-boosting
confidentiality 14, 25–6, 201–2; hypnotherapy 9; individual sessions 201–2; limits 25; and privacy 30, 31
conscious state 50, 115, 162; birthing plan 132; script 111, 162, 167, 213–15; *see also* subconscious mind; trance state
consent forms: hypnotherapy 23, 25–6; signing 21, 202; statements 25–6
Continued Professional Development (CPD) 4, 5, 10, 23, 29, 57
cooling down 16, 82, 85

Covid-19 pandemic 4, 13; and hypnobirthing 3; risk assessment 26n1
Crime and Disorder Act (1998) 26

dad: effect of miscarriage on 205; involvement in hypnobirthing 91–2; phobias 39; types 91
Data Protection Act (2018) 24, 26
death 15, 19, 122, 202; *see also* bereavement; loss; loss and bereavement
deposits, fees 33, 36
determination 16, 95, 96, 219, 225–6; promotion 19
Dick-Read: Grantly: Childbirth without Fear 4; Natural Childbirth 4
disability 9, 191; *see also* learning disabilities
discrimination 9
discriminatory abuse 10n11
distraction, script 194–5
diversity 9
divorce 203
Doel, M. 10
domestic abuse 6
domestic violence 8, 18
Domestic Violence, Crime and Victims Act (2004) 26
Douglas, T. 10
down breathing 62; bouncing ball 65; chocolate fountain 66; deep sea diving 66; the helicopter 68; raining round the lake 64–5; sledging on the hill 65; *see also* up breathing; up and down breathing

eating disorders 9
ego-boosting: script 222–4, 230–1; *see also* confidence building
ego strengthening 186
emotions, script 213–15
energising 82, 105
energy 99; gaining 105; lack of 84, 105, 219; restoring 17; soul as 205
equality 9
Equality Act (2010) 9
equipment, hypnobirthing group 31–2
Erickonsonian metaphors 12
evaluation 23–4; group questionnaire 24–5

fear(s): abused persons 8–9; assessment for 82; of blood, and assessment 39; for the future 228; and loss 202; of miscarriage 7; of the past 7, 193; script 182–3; *see also* phobias; feelings; worries
feelings 5; adoption of baby 208, 209; for the baby 7; concealing 216; flowerpot script 214–15; letting go of 210; negative 210, 219; positive 230; of regret 203; scripts 18, 19, 75, 102, 113, 121, 162, 167, 169, 177, 182; showing 213; stepdad 97; surrogate 39; trigger 202; visualisations 210

fees: deposits 33, 36; hypnobirthing group 33–4; hypnotherapy 34; individual sessions 41; *see also* payment

forced marriage 6, 8, 10n12

forms: of abuse 10n11; of consent 21, 202; evaluation 24

forward pacing 80, 145; scripts 16, 17, 18, 82, 133, 137

future, the: awareness of 198; changes for 229; development for 217; fears for 228; hope for 221; planning for 228; positivity 194, 198, 210; *see also* past, the

gay 4, 30

gender identity, and language change 10

General Data Protection Regulation (2018) 24, 26

Gestalt therapy 12

Graves: Katharine 4, 10n5, 61n4, 62, 68n1; work 58

grief 202; loss and bereavement 201; studies on 204n3; *see also* loss

grief therapy 201

group sessions 13, 21, 25, 62, 92, 127, 136

habit 7, 228

healing place: definition 17; script 104–7

health: emotional 48, 109; issues 38; *see also* mental health; physical health; wellbeing

health and safety 40, 80; *see also* lone working

home: bag packing 129; clothes for 130; individual sessions 40; running a business from 229; running a group from 30

home birthing (dad/birthing partner), script 18, 141, 154–6

home birthing (mum): questionnaire 135; scripts 18, 139, 151–4; visualisations 62

home visits 35, 39, 40–1

homelessness 9

hospital: goods needed in 130; packing a bag for 127, 128, 129; visiting 39; worries about 192

hospital journey (dad/birthing partner), script 141–4

hospital journey (mum): car 140; script 17, 18, 138–40

hospital setting (dad/birthing partner), script 148–50

hospital setting (mum), script 145–7

Human Rights Act (1998) 22

Hunter, R. 94n1

hypertension *see* blood pressure, high

hypno mat, imagination 16, 48

hypnobirthing: breathing exercises 58; and Covid-19 pandemic 3; dad involvement 91–2; language use 12–13; methods 4; popularity 3, 4; preparation 128–31

hypnobirthing group sessions: advertising 34; cost as deterrent 34; date and timing 34; equipment 31–2; fees 33–4; frequency and duration 32–3; key questions 36; lone working 35; programme 28–9; refreshments 32; risk assessment 35; running 27–8; screening 35; size 29–30; venue 30–1; visualisations 62–8; *see also* hypnobirthing individual sessions

hypnobirthing individual sessions: assessment 38–9; definition 37; fees 41; general topics to consider 37–8; home visits 40; package design 39; session length 39–40

hypnosis 5; benefits of 29, 37, 194; benefits therapy in 92; *see also* self-hypnosis

hypnotherapist: health and safety 5–6; issues to be aware of 8, 9–10; lone working 35, 40; problems encountered 5; registered 5; remote working 27; training 4–5

hypnotherapy: adults 39; and birthing 5; client-led 58; confidence building 184; confidentiality 9; consent form 23, 25–6; evaluation 23; fees 34; issues 7–8; and loss 208; positivity 193; practising 3; purpose 197; training suggestions 10

imagination: hypno mat 16, 48; power of 14; scripts 48–50, 89, 99, 119, 205–7; and subconscious mind 48

individual sessions 4, 16, 30, 162–9; assessment 21–3, 38; at home 40; breathing 58; confidentiality 201–2; fees 41; intended parents 16; issues 7, 37; refreshments 32; script 219–21; suitability 37; surrogacy 208; trance 92

intended parents: individual sessions 16; and surrogacy 10, 13, 19, 28, 38, 133, 203–4, 208

journal keeping, script 18, 162, 169

KGH method 4, 29, 57

Kubler-Ross, E., texts 204n3

language change, and gender identity 10

language use 7; client's preferred 13; hypnobirthing 12–13; positive 49; traditional 13; *see also* body language

learning disabilities, adults with 40

Leclaire method 29, 57

lesbians 4, 30

lifestyle: busy 57; healthy 95

lone working: hypnotherapists 35, 40; *see also* health and safety

loss: and angel's archway 19, 204; and fear 202; and hypnotherapy 208; in the past 15; triggers 201; typical situations 208; working through 202; *see also* death; grief; loss and bereavement loss and bereavement 10, 15; aspect of grief 201; learning about 201; major issue 201; and the past 201–2; potential to upset others 35; and pregnancy 202; script 205, 205–7; and secrets 201–2; types of 19; *see also* grief

mantras 90, 166, 187, 220, 222, 223, 231
Markus, A. 204
medical examinations 15, 19, 132, 191, 193; face-to-face sessions 13–14
memories 10; photographs 170; and pregnancy 15, 201; scripts 18, 19, 100, 169, 197; and subconscious mind 170
mental health 6, 22, 38; *see also* physical health
metaphors 12; scripts 20, 127, 130, 224, 227
miscarriage 91; disclosure, assessment 202; effect on dad 205; experience of 202; fear of 7; multiple 205, 207; script 19
modern slavery 8; studies 10n13
Mongan, Marie 58
Mongan method 4, 29, 57; examples 13
morning sickness: scripts 16, 17, 29, 38, 72, 75, 104, 106; *see also* nausea
motivation, script 16, 17, 95, 96

National Childbirth Trust (NCT) 34
nausea: scripts 16, 17, 72, 75, 106; *see also* morning sickness
needles, phobia 7
non-binary 4, 10, 13, 30, 220

obstacles, scripts 19, 219–21, 225
old wives' tales 184, 216
one-to-one sessions 39, 86, 164, 165, 166
O'Neill, Michelle Leclaire 4

parents *see* intended parents
Parkes: Colin Murray 201; texts 204n3
past, the: learning from 229; loss in 15; fears 7, 193; positive experiences 216; scripts 17, 18, 19, 119, 120–2, 197–8; and secrets 201–2; and the subconscious mind 121; *see also* future, the
past life 119, 121–2
payment 33–4, 36, 136; *see also* fees
pedalling: a bike, script 98–9; time away 17, 98
perpetrators of abuse *see* abusers
personal trainer, script 17, 97–8
phobias 5, 6, 25; assessment 38; needles 7; scripts 177–81; water 82, 100; *see also* fears; worries
photographs: memories 170; script 170–3; and the subconscious mind 171; suggestions 171
physical body, and the subconscious mind 111
physical health 22, 38, 95, 109
positivity, hypnotherapy 193

poverty 9, 34, 127; script 17
pregnancy: bad experiences 6; common fears 7–8; and memories 15, 201
privacy: and confidentiality 30, 31; and thoughts 37
Prigerson, H. 204
procedures 191, 192, 196; caesarean 193; clinical 4; forceps 193; medical 15, 19; stitches 193; unexpected 19

questionnaires: birthing plan 135; group evaluation 24–5

rape 6, 28, 132
refreshments 23, 36, 123, 132; hypnobirthing group 32
regression 8, 12, 32, 80; refusal to use 119; script 17, 119–23; techniques 119, 197
regret 15, 19, 23; feelings of 203; not knowing a child 204; of a surrogate 208
relationships: building 160; family 170; incestuous 6; loss of 203, 204; previous 91, 203, 204; safe 204; script 151, 227; unhappy 34
relaxation: and calmness 61; deep 45, 49, 121; groups 27; scripts 16–18, 45, 47, 51, 72, 92, 100, 111, 209; and the subconscious mind 134, 163; techniques 3; and trance state 14, 50, 54; true 47
remote working 14; hypnotherapist 27
risk assessment 22; contents 40; Covid-19 26n1; screening 35; written 40
room 30–1, 36, 90, 120, 138–9, 141–2; bath 100–3; birthing 70, 133–5, 145–50; function 183; home 151–2; message 162–3; therapy 82

safeguarding 11n14, 203; issues 9
Safeguarding Adults Board 9
Safeguarding Partnership, children 9
safe place 14, 51, 93; creation 48, 50, 92; scripts 16, 17, 119, 194
Sawdon, C. 10
scan 108–9, 171
scanner *see* body scanner
self-belief: building 184; development 19; lack of, script 222–4; promotion 20; script 222–3
self-confidence building, lack of, script 203, 224–5
self-doubt 5, 15, 18, 39, 220, 230
self-esteem 222, 224; low 5, 7, 15, 18, 39, 184, 203, 228
self-hypnosis: benefit 3, 231; practising 14, 45, 50, 51, 74, 90, 171, 230; scripts 16, 89–90, 194; and trance state 48
separation 203
secrets, and the past 201–2
sessions *see* group sessions; individual sessions

sexual abuse 6, 8, 10n10, 28, 132
slavery *see* modern slavery
sleeping problems, script 17, 116–18
solution-focused, methodologies 12
spirit guides 205
spirits, belief in 205
statements: consent forms 25–6;
    positive 166, 180–1
stepdad, feelings 97
stillbirth 7, 19, 91, 182, 202, 205, 207
stretch class, script 16, 96–7
subconscious mind 3, 5, 8; affect 7; and beliefs
    166; and imagination 48; memories 170; and
    the past 121; and photographs 171; and the
    physical body 111; power 95, 109, 111, 198,
    216; and relaxation 134, 163; scripts 17, 48,
    62, 109–10, 119, 133, 184–5, 194; and trance
    state 165; *see also* conscious state
suggestions: for hypnotherapy training
    10; photographs 171; positive thoughts
    102, 180–1
surrogacy 10, 203–4; individual sessions 208;
    and intended parents 10, 13, 19, 28, 38, 133,
    203–4, 208
surrogate: feelings 39; regrets of 208
survivors, of abuse 18, 100, 132, 184, 197

temperature: body 82; water 16, 72, 83, 85;
    weather 72
terminology 13
thoughts: and behaviour 102; intrusive 117,
    118, 196; negative 112, 187, 193, 194, 222;
    obsessive 5; positive 17, 18, 49, 165, 193,
    194, 220; and privacy 37; script 182
time: going faster 17, 82, 86, 95; passing 16;
    slowing down 99
trance; assessment for 50; individual
    sessions 92

trance state; benefits from 230; and relaxation
    14, 50, 54; and self-hypnosis 48; and
    subconscious mind 165, 167
transgender 4, 10, 13, 28
trauma, unexpected 15
traumatic incident 19

unexpected events, scripts 195–6
up breathing 62; bunches of balloons 63;
    butterfly house 64; cable car up the cliffs
    63–4; creatures in the sky 64; escalator 66–7;
    flying a kite 63; *see also* down breathing; up
    and down breathing
up and down breathing: the escalator 66–7;
    the helicopter 68; the lift 67; *see also* down
    breathing; up breathing

vaginal examination 134
venue 23, 30; equipment needed 31, 36;
    hiring 31, 36
victims, of abuse 8, 18, 20, 107, 185, 191, 193,
    197, 213
visualisations: feelings 210; home birthing
    (mum/birthing partner) 62; hypnobirthing
    group sessions 62–8

water; phobias 82, 100; script 82–6;
    temperature 16, 72, 83, 85
water park script 84–6
waterfall script 84
weight lifting, script 98
wellbeing 16; of baby 105; constituents 109;
    emotional 213; own 32, 48, 49, 90, 108–9;
    promotion 19, 29, 37; *see also*
    health
worries 7, 8, 15, 46, 52, 112; letting go of 123,
    130–1, 205, 206; scripts 17, 95, 177–81;
    see also concerns; fears; phobias

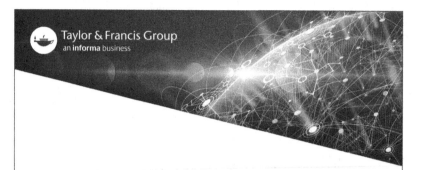

Printed in the United States
by Baker & Taylor Publisher Services